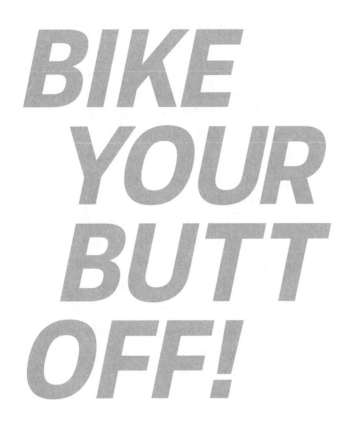

Also by Selene Yeager

The Active Calorie Diet (with the Editors of Prevention*)*

Get Fast!

The Prevention *Get Thin, Get Young Plan (with Bridget Doherty)*

The Men's Health *Big Book of 15-Minute Workouts*
(with the Editors of Men's Health*)*

Death Defiers (with the Editors of Men's Health*)*

Move a Little, Lose a Lot (with James Levine, MD, PhD)

Prevention*'s Complete Book of Alternative Nutrition*
(with the Editors of Prevention*)*

Prevention*'s New Foods for Healing*
(with the Editors of Prevention*)*

Ride Your Way Lean (with the Editors of Bicycling*)*

Selene Yeager's Perfectly Fit

The Show It Love Workout (with Kacy Duke)

30 Minutes a Day to a Healthy Heart (with the Editors of Reader's Digest*)*

What's with My Body? A Girls' Book of Answers
to Growing Up, Looking Good, and Feeling Great

The Women's Health *Big Book of 15-Minute Workouts*
(with the Editors of Women's Health*)*

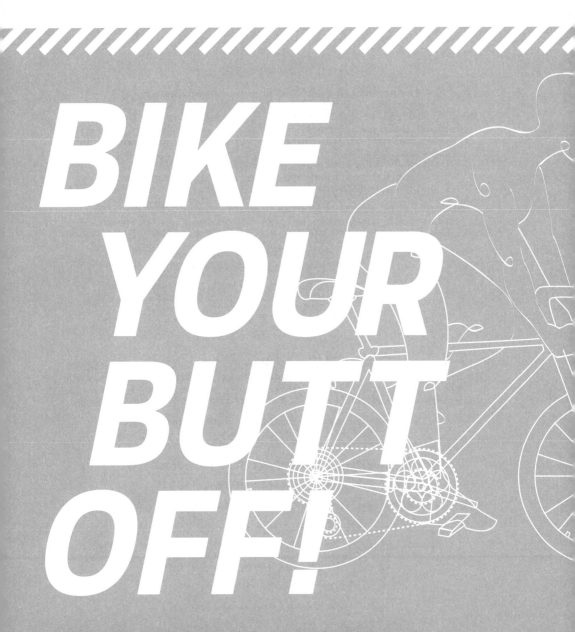

BIKE YOUR BUTT OFF!

A Breakthrough Plan to Lose Weight and Start Cycling (No Experience Necessary!)

Selene Yeager with Leslie Bonci, MPH, RD

Trade paperback and direct online hardcover editions published simultaneously by Rodale Inc. in March 2014.

© 2014 by Selene Yeager and Leslie Bonci

Photographs © 2014 by Tom MacDonald

Illustrations © Alix Nicholaeff

Rodale books may be purchased for business or promotional use or for special sales. For information, please write to: Special Markets Department, Rodale, Inc., 733 Third Avenue, New York, NY 10017

Bicycling is a registered trademark of Rodale Inc.

Printed in the United States of America

Rodale Inc. makes every effort to use acid-free ♾, recycled paper ♻.

Book design by Kara Plikaitis

Library of Congress Cataloging-in-Publication Data is on file with the publisher.

ISBN 978–1–60961–594–9 direct online hardcover

ISBN 978–1–60961–592–5 trade paperback

Distributed to the trade by Macmillan

2   4   6   8   10   9   7   5   3   1   hardcover

2   4   6   8   10   9   7   5   3   1   paperback

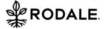

We inspire and enable people to improve their lives and the world around them.
rodalebooks.com

To my dad, for teaching me to ride.

CONTENTS

BECOMING A CYCLIST

IT'S A FUNNY THING. Nearly everyone can ride a bike. Nearly everyone has a bike. But relatively few people call themselves "cyclists," including many of those who ride regularly for fitness and fun. Worse, far too many people who have bikes don't use them as often as they'd like, despite the fact that cycling burns as many calories as jogging and more than twice as many as walking at even the fastest pace. Plus, cycling is easier on the joints and feels more like play than either jogging or walking.

Heck, there's a saying among medical (especially orthopedic) professionals that even when you can't walk or hobble, you can still ride a bike. You can do it if you have bad knees. You can do it if you have bad hips. You can do it if you can't run more than 5 feet. Nearly anyone of any fitness level can pedal a bike 5 or more miles. Cycling has been found to prevent weight gain (and boost fat loss), fight depression, and help stave off a host of health woes, including heart disease, cancer, and diabetes.

You'd think that with all bicycling has to offer, everyone and their Uncle Pete would be out there pedaling their hearts out. Yet, many who would like to and who would ultimately love the sport haven't tossed a leg over a bike in ages.

Why? Well, as a case in point I'll tell you about my friend Deb. She came to me a few years ago unhappy with the state of her waistline, which, now that she was well into her forties, was disappearing. She's never been one to go to the gym or exercise for the sake of exercise, but she does like outdoor activities like hiking. Living deep in the suburban DC sprawl, however, she didn't get to do that much anymore. She knew how much I loved riding and decided to give it a try.

She started making trips to the nearby store on her bike and going for rides on the local pedestrian path. She lost a pound or two, but before long the bike got relegated to a corner in her garage, tires as deflated as her once-pumped-up-motivation. What happened? The same thing that happens to so many would-be cyclists: No one ever told her *how to ride*. (And I don't mean putting your feet on the pedals and pushing them around.) No one told her how to get the most fun, challenge, pleasure, and fitness out of this remarkable machine—the bicycle.

Instead of flying around like a kid, tackling climbs, and swooping down hills, Deb pedaled hesitantly, sometimes feeling like she was fighting her bike rather than riding it. She pedaled aimlessly instead of purposefully. She got discouraged and lost interest.

It doesn't have to be that way. I've seen firsthand the transformative power of just a little know-how. Some simple instruction on how to shift, pedal, climb, brake, and corner can be the difference between riding year-round and hanging up your wheels for good. Knowing how to ride to best burn fat and tone muscles can turn even a short ride around town into a quality weight-loss workout. Mastering the art of riding also gives you the confidence to ride with others, which is one of cycling's most profound yet simple pleasures.

Newbies aren't the only ones who stand to benefit from some cycling instruction. I've spoken to and heard from countless riders who already love their bikes but still feel in the dark about the finer points of bike fit, pedaling, pacelining, and basic maintenance. All they need is a little nudge in the right direction to transform them from casual riders into *cyclists*.

Like Sherrie. When she first signed on to the Bike Your Butt Off! plan, she really liked to ride. But inexperience and nerves were holding her back from fully enjoying the cycling experience. "I don't know which levers shift which gears. And, well, this might be too much information, but I had to ice my girl parts after I rode this weekend, so I'm not doing something right," she told me upon our first meeting.

Just 4 weeks into the plan—1 month of receiving a little how-to—and Sherrie was sounding a whole lot like a cyclist: "I'm riding at least three times a week and learning so much from the drills, lessons, and interval training. I feel the training in places in my body where I don't normally feel it when I do indoor cycling, and I love that. I am getting much more confident on the bike outdoors and many of my fears (i.e., navigating an intersection with traffic lights and traffic, falling over because I'm clipped in to my pedals, riding in the rain, etc.) are going away and not holding me back. I talk about this project to everyone because I am so excited to be doing this."

And Jaime, who loves the idea of cycling and has started and stopped any number of times, had never before had the confidence to stick with it. "I love being on my bike now!" were the first words out of her mouth just 2 weeks into the plan. A couple weeks after that, she'd already dropped more than 5 pounds.

And Jim, probably the most experienced rider on our panel, was riding a lot but not losing much in the way of weight. After just 1 week he understood why. "I wasn't going hard enough often enough. That 3 minutes in Zone 4 is no fun. But it works," he wrote in an e-mail shortly after embarking on the BYBO plan. I guess it did. He shed 15 pounds.

If you're holding this book in your hands, chances are you share some of these feelings and experiences. Maybe you've seen the happy, fit, chatty cyclists cruising through your neighborhood and thought, "That looks fun," but didn't know how to get started. Maybe you loved riding as a kid but feel a little nervous about riding again after all these years. Or maybe you've tried gyms, running, Zumba, CrossFit, and/or other ways of getting fit, but they just didn't fit for you, and you wanted to give cycling a try.

Wherever you're coming from, you're in luck—and you've come to the right place. There is no better time than now to get on a bike. Cycling is enjoying a renaissance in this country. Gas prices have climbed to new heights, and they don't seem to be coming down anytime soon. Traffic is snarled. Increasingly, local governments are realizing the benefit of encouraging bicycling for both transportation and exercise and are building bike lanes and encouraging cyclists to take to the roads. This book will give you the confidence to join the record number of people who are saddling up and going out to ride!

Still not sure you're ready or willing to try your hand at cycling outdoors? Do you fancy yourself more suited to the Spin bike crowd? No worries! I've taught studio cycling for 17 years and worked with dozens of Spinning enthusiasts who aren't sure outdoor cycling is right for them, but they still want to learn how to take their indoor cycling to the next level. This book is for you, too! You'll find advice, plans, and workout routines to take the boredom out of stationary cycling, so you'll always have a fun and effective workout to do at the gym, at a hotel, or in your own rec room, where your stationary bike has been gathering dust. (And if you have a change of heart and decide to ride outdoors, you have a whole set of plans for that, too—two books in one!)

Nearly half the test panel were gym goers, runners, and other fitness enthusiasts who had bikes and were curious about riding, but primarily wanted to learn what to do on a stationary bike (either in their home or at the gym) to lose weight. Their experience with this plan was overwhelmingly positive.

"I just loved having specific workouts and drills to do," said Crystal Reese, who did the BYBO plan with her husband, Russ. "I got stronger almost immediately once I understood how to push myself and recover properly."

For even more options, I'll show riders—both indoor and outdoor—how to turn their beater bikes into highly effective indoor weight-loss and fitness machines for the cold, dark months when the opportunities to get outside dwindle from slim to nonexistent.

BIKE YOUR BUTT BEAUTIFUL

Yes, the book is called *Bike Your Butt Off!*, but you know that won't literally happen. What *will* literally happen is you will bike your butt *beautiful*. Cycling is so good for getting fit because it puts all those large, calorie-burning muscles in your lower body to work, toning and trimming your quads, hamstrings, calves, and of course your glutes! Cycling also offers numerous unique health benefits.

STEADY, SUSTAINABLE FAT LOSS. If you're looking for a quick weight-loss fix, you're in the wrong place. You'll lose weight—a number of panelists lost 10 to 15 pounds. But those pounds will peel off at a reasonable, steady, and, most important, *sustainable* pace. Even at a recreational pace of about 13 to 15 miles per hour, you burn around 500 to 600 calories in one hour, or about 4,000 calories per week—enough to burn off more than a pound a week if you ride about an hour a day. Cycling also sparks metabolic and physiological changes that turn you into a highly efficient fat and carbohydrate burner all day long.

It starts in your legs. Cycling builds a giant web of hundreds of thousands of capillaries throughout your legs, which means you can deliver more oxygen-rich blood to your working muscles. At the same time, your mitochondria—the energy-producing furnaces in your muscle cells—get bigger, so they can use the increased influx of oxygen to burn more fat and produce more energy. Research shows that when sedentary people start riding just 30 minutes per day, five times a week, their capillary per fiber ratio (i.e., the number of blood vessels per muscle fiber) in their quads soared by 40 percent, their mitochondria got 15 percent denser, and the amount of oxygen their legs could use during exercise shot up 13 percent after just *8 weeks*.

Cycling also coaxes your body to continue burning fat and calories for hours after you've racked your bike. For one, while you're riding, your LPL (lipoprotein lipase, a fat-shuttling enzyme) activity goes into high gear, and it remains elevated for a full 30 hours after you've stopped riding. After a ride, your body—hence your metabolism—is still revved up, working to replenish and (if you worked really hard that day) repair your muscles. As you get fitter and stronger, your basal metabolic rate (BMR)—the calories you burn by just living—goes up. Getting just 30 to 45 minutes of exercise most days of the week can boost your BMR and keep it in the up position permanently.

The end result is fat loss—and lots of it. Even better, you'll lose it first where you want it least, in your belly, where it smothers your organs and leads to heart disease, diabetes, and other diseases. In one study of 24 men and women with diabetes, those who biked 45 minutes three times a week for 8 weeks decreased their visceral fat (the deep belly fat) by a staggering 48 percent.

As you move further into the program (and turn up that pace a little higher), you'll fry fat even faster. Cyclists who pepper their regular rides with some fast-paced intervals burn $3\frac{1}{2}$ times more calories than their one-speed counterparts. And they have more fun, too!

HEART HEALTH. Cycling is a cardiovascular activity, so it goes without saying it makes your heart stronger and healthier. Exercise like cycling also makes your skeletal muscle more insulin sensitive, so you're better able to control your blood sugar level—something scientists now know is essential for clear arteries and good heart health. The overall protective impact cycling has on your heart is pretty impressive. The British Medical Association reports that cycling just 20 miles a week—which you'll be doing on the Bike Your Butt Off! plan—slashes your risk of coronary heart disease *in half* compared with staying sedentary.

BIGGER, HEALTHIER BRAIN. Neuroscientists think of exercise as Miracle-Gro for the brain because it's a powerful, neuron-building stimulant that works remarkably fast. Exercise that raises your heart rate, like cycling, dramatically increases the production of nitric oxide (a potent vasodilator) and neurotrophins (growth factors) such as brain-derived neurotrophic factor and a protein aptly named noggin, which promotes stem cell division and new brain cell formation.

In one study, neuroscientists examined the brains of formerly sedentary people who started a moderate aerobic exercise program. After just 3 months of regular activity, the subjects had the brain volumes of men and women 3 years younger; that increased volume equals better cognitive performance. In a joint study by the University of Illinois and the University of Pittsburgh, researchers found that volunteers who were physically fit had larger hippocampi (the region of the brain that controls memory) and performed 40 percent better on memory tests.

The end result is that cycling will give you better, sharper memory skills, stronger concentration ability, more fluid thinking and reasoning, and greater problem-solving abilities. All this brain building also protects you from age-related cognitive decline and Alzheimer's disease and other dementias.

SLEEP LIKE A BABY. It's hard to overstate the importance of sleep. Your body and brain heal while you rest. Without enough sleep, your hormone levels (especially stress hormones) get out of whack, and you're more likely to overeat and gain weight, as well as have more mood disorders and lowered immunity. In one of the most striking studies on the subject, the sleep habits and body-weight trends of 68,000 women were studied over a period of 16 years. The researchers found that those who slept only 5 hours a night were 32 percent more likely to gain 33 pounds or more over the course of the study compared with their peers who slept 7 hours a night. Regular aerobic exercise like cycling promotes quality sleep even among those who struggle to get their shut-eye. In a study by researchers at the Stanford University School of Medicine, previously sedentary insomnia suffers who started cycling just 20 to 30 minutes every other day reduced the amount of time it took to fall asleep by half and increased their total sleep time by nearly an hour.

MILES OF SMILES. You rarely see someone finish a ride grumpy. To the contrary—they're usually grinning from ear to ear. Cycling lifts your spirits—nearly immediately. In one study from Bowling Green State University, researchers found that as little as 10 minutes of cycling improved the mood in a group of volunteers compared with their peers who just relaxed for the same amount of time.

Undoubtedly, part of cycling's mood magic results from its stress-blasting effects. Exercise, such as pedaling a bike, burns off excess adrenaline you've built up during meetings with the boss and the hassles of the day; it also slows the production of the stress hormone cortisol, which has been linked to weight gain. Cycling also boosts the production of feel-good hormones like serotonin and dopamine. For some people, it can work as well as antidepressants. One study at the University of Southern Mississippi found that men and women suffering from generalized anxiety disorder who started doing just 20-minute exercise sessions three times a week reported significantly less anxiety and general fearfulness after just two workouts. Even better, research shows that by doing regular vigorous exercise, you're less likely to develop anxiety disorders and depression to begin with.

A TRIED-AND-TRUE PROGRAM

To help riding enthusiasts and aspiring riders of every stripe and experience level learn how to ride like cyclists and reap all the rewards the sport has to offer, we crafted the plan you are holding in your hands—a 12-week, step-by-step guide to really learning how to ride.

The focus of this program is fitness—that means making you faster, stronger, and leaner. To do that you need to master riding hard against resistance (like uphills), pedaling with blazing fast speed (like sprinting), and holding a brisk pace for longer periods.

Each week's workout will home in on a key cycling fitness and/or skill element to keep your progress rolling along (pun intended). The workouts are designed to challenge your muscles and cardiovascular system in a relatively short time. So give them your full attention and effort. You'll be rewarded with bigger calorie burn. Food for thought: Riding at a fairly leisurely 10 miles per hour burns about 500 calories an hour. Ratchet it up to 15 miles per hour, and you burn nearly 200 more.

For outdoor riders, this means mastering the machine—braking, shifting, steering, pedaling, and so on—as well as learning how to mete out your efforts to get the most effective fitness-building, fat-burning workout from your ride. To work properly, we have to start from the ground up. So the plan may start at an instructional level that feels a bit too simple if you've been riding for a while. Please go through the drills anyway. I bet you'll be surprised at what you learn.

Spinning bike workouts will incorporate strength-training moves within the workout. Outdoor riders will be doing some core work as well, but you should do the moves at another convenient time (since you're not going to get off your bike and do them on the pavement).

For inside riders, the goal is similar: teaching you how to get the most out of that stationary or Spin bike in the gym or your rec room, so you actually enjoy riding it and reap real fitness benefits without having it feel like a chore. Ultimately I'd love to see you transition to trying some outside riding. But it's perfectly okay to start the course indoors.

Each chapter in this book represents a week in the workout plan. So, every week, you'll find new Skill Drills, cycling advice, and workouts for both indoor and outdoor riding, as well as some bonus stretching and strengthening exercises. Because exercise doesn't work in a vacuum, you'll also be given eating recommendations. Bike Your Butt Off! is not a diet. And we want you to fuel your rides, so no spartan, counting-the-days–until–you-can-eat-again diets here. Here's what to expect each week.

THE CYCLING PLAN. You'll be cycling 4 days per week. Three of those rides will include structured drills to help build your fitness, strength, stamina, and confidence (as well as burn fat and calories, of course). One day per week will be a pleasure cruise. If you can do more, fantastic. If you can manage only three, simply work in an extra day of cross-training. Everyone is strapped for time, so this program aims to teach you how to get the most out of workouts in less than an hour. If you generally ride outside, but can't get out on a particular day, use your trainer if you have one. Or do the Inside Ride option.

THE EATING PLAN. Notice, "plan" not "diet." Our goal is to have you find the perfect fit, so just like your bike, you need to fit your eating to your own requirements, lifestyle, energy expenditure, and so forth. And it is not going to be coasting—there are lots of uphill climbs—but just as the bike wheels don't revolve without your effort, the same is true of eating. If you want to be lean, fit, and healthy, you need to make the effort in choosing what, when, and how much you eat on a daily basis.

To be perfectly clear, weight loss is not easy. Weight loss is not a slide; it's more like steps. It doesn't happen in one smooth, fell swoop, but rather bit by bit, with some pauses along the way. Losing weight should not be about denial and deprivation, and so the focus here is going to be on what you *can* and *should* do. And, remember, we cannot make you do it—that is up to you. We're just here to guide, advise, teach, and motivate.

On that note, since we all have different food likes, dislikes, hungry times, and busy hours, eating cannot be one-size-fits-all. Many clients adopt an all-or-nothing approach when it comes to eating (no carbs, no fat, no white foods), and when they don't follow their "plan," they feel guilty or, worse yet, give up and go back to old habits and food choices. We really don't want that to happen, which is why we will give you weekly goals, tips, and strategies for the 3 months of the BYBO program. Yes, we'll talk about ingredients and specific foods, too, but we really want you to take a critical look at your current habits and the changes you need to make. Eating needs to become a mental exercise, not just a physical one. You have a chance to try out some new foods and new habits, and at the end of the 12 weeks, you decide what you keep and what you don't. Sound reasonable? We thought so.

To put this plan to the test, we recruited a Bike Your Butt Off! test panel of men and women just like you—busy folks with families and full-time jobs and all the general chaos and responsibilities that come with living life. The group was split pretty evenly between indoor and outdoor riders, with a few of the panelists opting to mix it up and do both.

As you've seen from some of their words and stories above, they did well—very well. You'll find more of their stories—as well as some of their own hard-earned advice—sprinkled throughout the book.

WHO WE ARE

Your coach for this training session is Selene Yeager (that's me!). I am a licensed USA Cycling coach, certified personal trainer, studio cycling instructor, and semiprofessional mountain bike racer for Team CF. I've been dishing out training advice as *Bicycling* magazine's "Fit Chick" since 1999. I am also the primary writer of the book. Cycling is more than a sport for me. It's a way of life. My bike has taken me countless wonderful places in this world and in my life, and I am over the moon when I can help other people get on bikes and pedal off on their own great adventures. I'm very happy to help you get off the ground for yours.

I am joined by world-renowned sports dietitian Leslie Bonci, MPH, RD, CSSD, LDN (that's a lot of credentials right there!), who works at the University of Pittsburgh Medical Center. Her clients range from the average person who wants to lose weight to pro athletes who play for the Steelers, Penguins, and Pirates. Leslie may work with superstars, but she has both feet planted firmly on the ground in the real world. She works long hours, exercises almost every day during the week, and buys her food to feed her family from a regular grocery store like everyone else. She's here to help you make better choices and fuel your body with the healthiest (and tastiest) fare, *not* to make eating a joyless chore.

That's the plan in a nutshell. Turn the page, and let's get ready to roll.

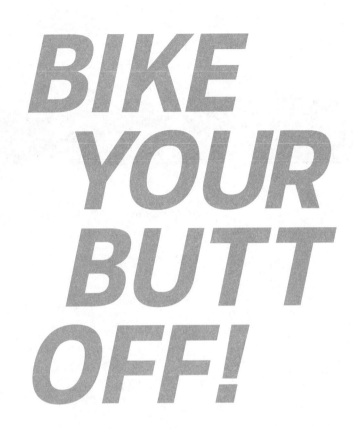

CHAPTER 1

GET YOUR WHEELS SPINNING

THE PURPOSE OF THIS book is to make cycling fun, easy, and effective for everyone. We're not concerned about your current skill level or whether or not you have all the latest and greatest cycling gear. Once you become hooked, you can run out and empty your wallet on a sexy carbon bike with the works, if you'd like. But right now, you just need the bare minimum—a bike that you can ride (even if it's a stationary one), the desire to get fit, and the willingness to learn a few new skills (on the bike and in the kitchen—we'd like to lose some weight after all!). Seriously, that's it.

Before we get to the fun stuff—the riding!—let's make sure you have those essentials covered. This chapter will be one of the longest in the book—but don't be daunted. There is a lot to discuss right out of the gate, but it's not complicated, I promise.

GATHER YOUR GEAR

First things first. Let's take a look at your bike. If you'll be using a bike you already have, you'll want to take a few simple steps to be sure it's ready to roll (literally and figuratively).

WHAT TYPE OF BIKE WILL YOU RIDE?

The type of bike that you have defines the type of riding experience you will have. Road bikes handle differently than mountain bikes, which handle differently than hybrids. Though you can use any bike while following the Bike Your Butt Off! plan, knowing what you're riding will help you get the most from your workouts.

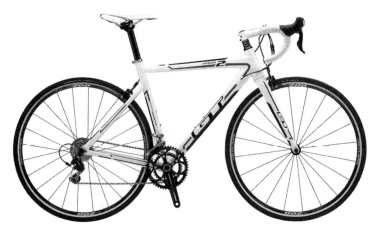

DEFINING FEATURES. As the name implies, road bikes are specially constructed to ride on hard surfaces like pavement. They are traditionally built for speed (i.e., racing), so you'll generally find curved "drop" handlebars, which allow you to tuck into a low aerodynamic position, as well as skinny tires that lessen the amount of rolling resistance you have on the road. Bikes in this category range in price from $500 to $10,000 (seriously) and include everything from featherweight pro racing bikes like you see in the Tour de France to sturdy touring bikes that can carry racks and packs.

HOW IT RIDES. Quick, efficient, and responsive. Of all the bikes you can ride, road bikes will likely give you the most speed for your pedal power. They also tend to be easy to maneuver, which is a good thing, but can make some new riders feel a little nervous because the bike responds to their every movement and the tires are very narrow.

HOW TO BIKE YOUR BUTT OFF! ON IT. Road bikes are great for biking your butt off because they are up to the task of going for long rides, climbing hills, and pedaling hard and fast. If you'll be doing the Bike Your Butt Off! plan on a road bike, pay special attention to all the Skill Drills involving shifting, braking, cornering, and pedaling. You'll be using them all a whole lot on a road bike, and the better you master them, the more fun you'll have and the fitter you'll become.

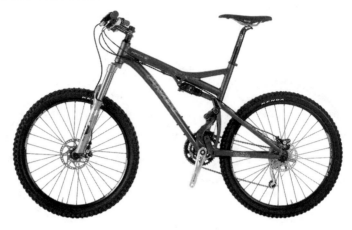

DEFINING FEATURES. Mountain bikes are designed to excel where the sidewalk ends. So you'll find features like big, knobby tires and generally some suspension system (shock absorbers in the front and/or the rear) that allows you to roll over rough terrain with relative ease. They also come equipped with flat handlebars and position the rider in a more upright than bent-forward position. These, too, come in a very wide price range, from a few hundred to several thousand dollars. Unless you're going to be doing serious off-road mountain biking, a lower-priced model will do just fine.

HOW IT RIDES. Stable and fun. These confidence-inspiring steeds make you feel like you can ride over anything. Curbs and potholes and roots and rocks? No problem. Mountain bikes don't roll as quickly on asphalt as road bikes, but they still go plenty fast and are very versatile machines.

HOW TO BIKE YOUR BUTT OFF! ON IT. The nice part about using a mountain bike for the Bike Your Butt Off! plan is you have plenty of options for where to ride. If you don't feel comfortable on the street, you can easily do your workouts on a bridle path or trail. Although *Bike Your Butt Off!* isn't a guide to hard-core mountain biking, pay attention to the Skill Drills like shifting, pedaling, braking, and climbing that will help you get the most pleasure—and fitness—from your riding.

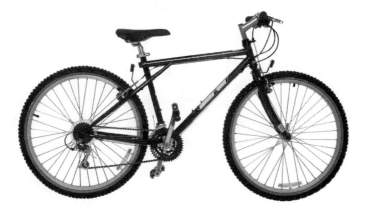

DEFINING FEATURES. A hybrid bike looks like the kind of bike you'd probably draw a picture of as a kid. They generally put the rider in a fairly upright position, have flat bars, and have medium-width tires that roll smoothly and briskly on pavement but are wide enough to provide stability on gravel paths and bumpy dirt roads. They generally run in middle-of-the-road price range, from $400 to $1,200, depending on the quality of the materials and components used.

HOW IT RIDES. Brisk and comfortable. Hybrid bikes are not speed demons, but they still roll comfortably at a nice clip. These bikes often inspire confidence in novice riders because the riding position is less "racy" than a traditional road bike, and because there's no suspension, they tend to be less complicated than a true mountain bike.

HOW TO BIKE YOUR BUTT OFF! ON IT. A hybrid is a great Bike Your Buff Off! tool because you can ride it comfortably pretty much anywhere, from your neighborhood streets to smooth dirt bike trails. They also are nice commuting and errand-running machines. You can do all the prescribed workouts on your hybrid. As with road and mountain bikes, to get the most out of your hybrid, pay attention to the Skill Drills like shifting, pedaling, braking, and climbing.

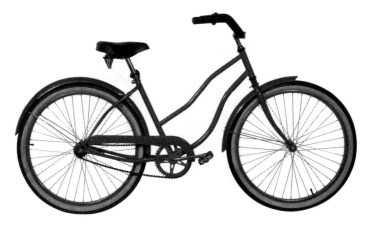

DEFINING FEATURES. These bikes are built to let you sip a latte while you spin down the road. They have wide seats and high handlebars that put the rider in a very erect position. They tend to have wide tires for great stability. They also tend to be heavier than other types of bikes.

HOW IT RIDES. Steady and easy. As the name implies, they are not designed to sprint to any finish lines or tackle technical trails—they are meant to cruise. They also tend to be very simple to operate, since they often have fewer gears than other bikes, and you're meant to hop on them and go.

HOW TO BIKE YOUR BUTT OFF! ON IT. You can do the Bike Your Butt Off! workouts on your beach cruiser, but it will be trickier than it would be on one of the other bike types mentioned. Simply put, a cruiser is designed mostly for pleasant pedaling on flat ground. They don't have the geometry, gearing, or saddle position that lets you easily tackle steep climbs or descents. That's not to say that you need to run out and buy a new bike. But you will likely need to tweak your workouts a bit, especially in terms of terrain. For instance, you won't need a very steep hill to get a great workout on your cruiser, you'll have fewer gears to experiment with in the shifting sections, and your overall pedaling cadence will likely be slower.

TUNE IT UP

If you are riding a bike that's been sitting idle for more than a few months (years?), take it to a bike shop and get a tune-up. Cables rust. Rubber rots. All sorts of deterioration can happen over time that can make your bike not only less than pleasurable to ride, but also perhaps unsafe. You want your bike to shift smoothly, brake reliably, and roll smoothly, and a tune-up is affordable insurance that it will. It can also be nice to have a relationship with the workers in your local bike shop, who can be a valuable resource for finding rides and riding partners in your area.

Are you in the market to buy a new bike? If so, consider the points made about each bike in the section above. Before you buy, take some time to consider where you'll ride and what kind of riding you'll be doing.

DO A SEAT CHECK

Before you embark on the BYBO plan, do yourself a favor and check the height of your seat (technically known as the saddle). New riders often ride with their saddles too low, likely because they want to be able to plant both feet on the ground when seated. This position makes it very hard to generate much power, since you never get proper leg extension, and also is hard on your knees and can lead to an overuse injury.

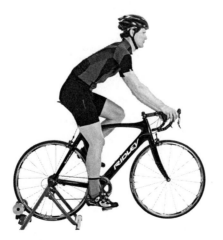

You should only be able to touch the ground on your tiptoes in the seated position. When pedaling in the seated position, your leg should be nearly straight, with just about a 25-degree bend in your knee, when your foot is at the bottom of the pedal stroke (the lowest position). This position also applies to an indoor Spin bike. Conversely, if your leg gets fully extended and your hips rock when you pedal, your saddle is too high. That's far less common. But give yourself a check and make sure the height is just right.

COVER YOUR TOP AND YOUR BOTTOM

Glance through the window of any bike shop, and you'll discover a whole new universe of clothing and gear available to the budding cyclist. It all serves a purpose, but that doesn't mean you *need* it all to ride a bike. Two items I would encourage you to invest in right out of the gate are a helmet and a comfortable pair of cycling shorts.

A helmet is nonnegotiable. It doesn't matter how safe a rider you are or how well you handle a bike. Stuff happens. Even on a path through a park where you don't have to worry about traffic, there are dogs, squirrels, pedestrians, and any number of things that can cause a tumble. Why tempt fate with your brain? Helmets today are comfortable and affordable. Any helmet sold in the United States must meet the US Consumer Product Safety Commission standard (as indicated by the CPSC sticker inside the helmet). Once you find one you like in your price range, strap it on every time you ride. It should sit low and evenly across your forehead, the side straps should form a V under your earlobes, and you should be able to slide two fingers between the chinstrap and your skin.

You can ride without special shorts. I know plenty of people who do so, and I myself did for years. But I promise, once you try a pair, you'll never go for a long ride without them again. Cycling specific shorts have padding (called a chamois) where you need it most—under your rear and tender nether regions. They increase your riding comfort exponentially. We highly recommend buying a pair from your local sporting goods store if you don't own any. While you certainly don't need a helmet for indoor cycling, cycling shorts are still a great idea. Oh, and just so you're in the know—cycling shorts are made to be worn *without* underwear; nothing screams "Newbie!" like visible underwear lines.

FIND THE TIME AND PLACE

If there is one downside to cycling as a mode of fitness, it is that it is not quite as convenient as running or walking. It takes a bit more time to get out and ride than it does to walk out the door. So it's important to make blocking out that time a priority.

You've heard this advice before, but it works: Schedule your bike rides like you would any other meeting. Write them down on your calendar, plug them into your iPhone, put them on your computer iCalendar—however you schedule appointments, *do it.* Also, tell the key people in your life about your plans and ask for their help. If you want to ride after work but usually pick up groceries at that time, see if your spouse can do it on those days. Or take a page from Crystal and Russ Reese's book and plan your workouts *with* your spouse. As Crystal told me in Week 3 of the BYBO test-drive period, "Russ and I are really enjoying ourselves; it's nice to *have to* spend time together."

Make this your "must have" time and protect it like you would an important meeting or a night on the town. A key part of this plan is building consistency. You want to get in the habit of getting on your bike regularly. If you get nothing else out of the program, you've won. This might mean that sometimes the dishes have to wait or the laundry goes unsorted for the day. That's okay. Those daily to-dos always get done. You are the priority for the next 12 weeks as you build new healthy-lifestyle habits.

As for where to ride, consider the options closest and most convenient to you first. Do you have a rail trail, park, or other greenway nearby? They're perfect places to begin. Even simpler is riding around your neighborhood or on quiet back roads. Still uncertain? Stop by your local bike shop and ask

(continued on page 12)

GET TO KNOW YOUR BIKE

Every bike has some basic components that allow you to pedal, steer, stop, and otherwise pilot it down the road. Here are the basic parts you should know.

❶ **HANDLEBARS.** They can be straight, curved, or somewhere in between. As the name implies, the handlebars ("bars" for short) are what you hold onto to control the bike.

❷ **SHIFTERS.** Generally located on the handlebars (except on older road bikes, where they are on the frame), the shifters allow you to change gears. The shift levers on the left side generally control the front derailleur, which moves the chain from chainring to chainring for big shifts like going from ground level to a climb. The right shifter generally controls the back derailleur, used for more subtle shifts. Shift levers can be levers that you push or, in some cases, dials that you rotate around the handlebar grips.

❸ **DERAILLEURS.** The front derailleur guides the chain from chainring to chainring. The rear derailleur guides the chain up and down the gears on the rear cassette.

❹ **BRAKE LEVERS.** On your bars next to (or sometimes integrated with) the shifters, these are the levers you pull to slow down and/or stop the bike. The left brake lever generally works the front brake; the right works the rear. In the case of cruiser bikes, you may not have levers, but rather coaster brakes that you activate by pedaling backward.

❺ **BRAKE.** The mechanism holding the pads that squeeze part of your wheel (generally the rim or a special braking disc attached to the center of the wheel) to slow down and stop the bike.

❻ **CHAINRINGS.** The big gears on the front of the drivetrain (the entire mechanism that propels your bike when you pedal). You'll generally have two or three, the biggest being the "hardest" and the smallest being the "easiest."

❼ **CASSETTE.** The smaller gears in the rear of the drivetrain. On the cassette, the bigger gears are actually the "easiest" and the smaller ones the "hardest."

❽ **WHEELS.** You need two for your bike to roll. They consist of rims (the skinny or fat outer part that the tires sit on), hubs (the center part that attaches to the bike), and spokes (the skinny rails that hold it all together). Not surprisingly, lighter wheels roll faster.

❾ **TIRES.** These are the parts that make contact with the ground. They can be smooth, knobby, or somewhere in between depending on the kind of bike and the surfaces you ride on. Inside the tire is an inner tube that you inflate with air.

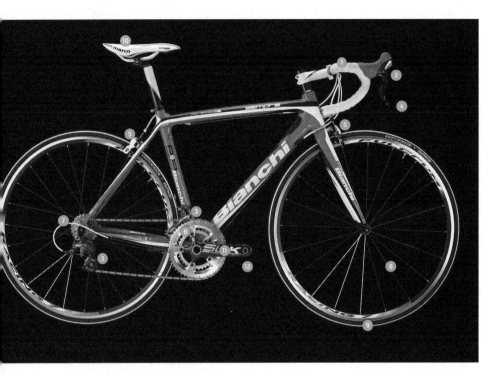

SADDLE. The part you sit on, which makes it one of the most important parts of your bike. Many new riders don't know that you can buy a different saddle or swap saddles if you're buying a new bike. So if you're not comfortable on yours, you can shop around to find one that is the perfect fit for you (more on that to come).

CRANKS. The arms that attach the pedals to your bike.

PEDALS. The platforms you place your feet on. This bike is shown with no pedals. Many cyclists replace the stock pedals with ones of their own preference. Some pedals are flat; others are special varieties called clipless pedals, which attach to a cleat that is fastened onto cycling-specific shoes. Most cycling enthusiasts eventually opt for clipless pedals because it maximizes power throughout the pedal stroke and increases the efficiency (and enjoyment) of the ride. That said, flat pedals work just fine.

where they ride. Or simply Google "bike paths and [the name of your area]." You'll likely be surprised by how many options are available to you.

Also consider taking your bike to work (maybe even riding it there if that's possible). Page 47 provides instructions for removing the front wheel, which makes nearly any bike fit neatly across the backseat of a car. Then go for a spin on your lunch hour. Trust me, nothing makes you happier or more productive at work than a midday spin in the sun.

Finally, keep all your cycling stuff in one convenient location, so you don't have to go hunting for your helmet or shorts when you want to ride. That's especially important if you plan on riding in the mornings, when having your stuff scattered throughout the house may tempt you to hit snooze and roll over rather than to get up and ride.

GEARING UP FOR HEALTHY EATING

So you have your bike all ready to embark on the exercise part of the BYBO plan. Now it's time to gear up to tackle the other half of the fitness–weight loss equation: food. Leslie wants you to bring your training into the kitchen. The first step? Start doing more of your food prep at home.

As a culture, we are eating out, taking out, and grabbing-and-going more than ever. It's convenient, yes. But it's also a key reason for our ever-expanding waistlines. The food that you get at restaurants is often loaded with hidden calories in the forms of starch, sugar, and fat. That's why taking charge of your health and your weight starts with taking charge of your food.

We don't want you to give up your day job or shortchange your rides to spend long hours in the kitchen, but it is our hope that over the next few months, you'll unleash your inner chef and spend some time cooking. Studies have shown that the satisfaction derived from eating is not from just the hand-to-mouth activity, but also the food prep. Having an active kitchen means a lot of cutting, chopping, mixing, blending, stirring—upper-body activity to complement your lower-body cycling work.

So let's take a peek inside your kitchen. You'll need a few basic tools to get the job done. Here are a few suggestions. You likely don't have all of these—and that's okay. Dig out and/or dust off the ones that you do, so making more of your meals at home is as quick and convenient as going through the drive-through or eating out.

- **TOASTER OVEN:** for fish, chicken, homemade pizza, and more

- **SLOW COOKER:** for soups, stews, sauces, oatmeal

- **RICE COOKER:** for no-fuss grains; can also steam veggies

- **MICROWAVE:** for reheating all those great dishes

- **BLENDER:** for smoothies

- **COUNTERTOP GRILL OR STOVETOP GRILL PAN:** for cooking meats and eggs

BIKE YOUR BUTT OFF! WORKOUT BASICS

Time to get started! But before we get to your Week 1 workouts, let's lay the general groundwork for the workouts. As mentioned earlier, every week you'll have Skill Drills designed to help you improve a specific facet of riding as well as a fitness-based workout.

The cycling workouts will be prescribed by time and intensity level. You'll also find four core moves to build abdominal and back strength (and flatten your abs to boot!), as well as a handful of stretches, which will directly increase your cycling comfort and improve your performance. Everything can be done in about an hour's time. Here are some general guidelines.

* You can do any of the workouts on back-to-back days. But recognize that without a break, such as a cross-training day or a day off, between some of the harder workouts, you may be a bit more fatigued.

* You can do BYBO and Core Workouts every day if you'd like, but shoot for at least 3 days a week.

* Stretch in the mornings or evenings (or both) to stay limber.

* Stay active on days off the bike. Go for a walk. Take a yoga class. Swim. Whatever appeals to you. Just get up and move for at least 30 minutes. Your body was made to move, and it feels and performs best when you exercise daily.

SAMPLE WEEKLY SCHEDULE *WEEK 1*

MONDAY	TUESDAY	WEDNESDAY	THURSDAY	FRIDAY
BYBO and Core Workouts	Off or Crosstrain	BYBO and Core Workouts	Crosstrain	Off or Crosstrain

SATURDAY	SUNDAY
BYBO and Core Workouts	Pleasure cruise

INTENSITY-LEVEL GUIDELINES

Here are the effort levels that you'll be aiming for when you pedal. Intensity levels are very subjective and are affected by your current fitness level. Beginners will not have to go as fast to hit the appropriate intensity level, but will still get similar benefits. As you become more fit, you will find that you need to increase the intensity to be working out at that same level. That's a good sign, showing that your heart and body are becoming better conditioned. Most important, listen to your body, and ride at a pace that's appropriate for you.

ZONE	INTENSITY	HOW IT FEELS	SPEED ESTIMATES (MPH)*
1	Easy	Nearly effortless pedaling. Light tension in your legs. Aerobic breathing, but no huffing and puffing.	8–12
2	Moderate	Pedaling with purpose. More (but manageable) tension in your legs. Steady, heavier, rhythmic breathing; can still carry on short conversation.	12–16
3	Hard	Jamming. Legs are working hard. Breathing hard. Talking impossible.	16–20
4	Max	Full throttle. Pedaling at full tilt. Huffing and puffing. Can't keep it up long.	20+

These are only very rough speed estimates. So many factors (bike type, terrain, wind, weather, etc.) affect speed, it's impossible to take them all into consideration. Some people like to use a bike computer to track their speed. Others do not. You don't even need one. In any event, please don't get too hung up on the numbers. Effort is what counts.

ON THE BIKE: LET'S GET ROLLING

This week we start with the basics—starting, stopping, and scanning for traffic. If you've been riding for a while, these may seem really basic, but believe it or not, these are essential skills that even some seasoned riders could use some practice in perfecting.

// **SKILL DRILL:** Starting, Scanning, and Stopping

STARTING. In a parking lot or on a safe, open stretch of road, practice starting and rolling out smoothly. As soon as you're rolling, stop, put a foot down, and start again, aiming for no wobbling. Do this 5 times. (It helps to start in a slightly harder gear rather than an easier one, so you can get some momentum quickly.)

Still feeling wobbly? Here are some tips for smooth, seamless starts.

STRADDLE THE BIKE. Swing a leg over the bike and straddle the top tube with both feet flat on the ground. Use a foot to turn your pedals backward and place the pedal for your dominant foot forward and slightly up. (Your lead foot is simply the one you feel most comfortable pushing off with, usually the same as your dominant hand.)

SQUEEZE THE BRAKES, PUT DOMINANT FOOT ON THE LEADING PEDAL. This is the ready position. First, scan over your shoulder for traffic (a good habit to get into). Then . . .

RELEASE AND PUSH OFF. Let go of the brakes and push down with your lead foot as you simultaneously push off the ground with the other foot, lifting yourself up and onto the saddle.

PLANT SECOND FOOT AND PEDAL. Place your other foot on its pedal and start pedaling, shifting your rear into position at the back of the saddle as you start rolling.

SCANNING. After practicing a few starts from a stopped position, start again. As you're rolling, scan over your left shoulder as if looking for cars. The bike should not veer left. Perform five scans to each side, working to keep the bike steady and moving in a straight line during each.

STOPPING. Finally, hone your stopping skills. Your front brake contains about 70 percent of your stopping power, so it's very effective. Just remember that stopping your front wheel too hard and fast makes you very unstable very quickly, so use a soft touch with it.

You'll discover that as you squeeze the brakes, your bike slows down but your body keeps going, sending your weight forward over the front wheel and making it difficult to steer. Counter this effect by shifting your weight back on the saddle as you squeeze the brake levers.

Shifting your weight back is especially important when you're stopping on a decline. New riders often don't like to go downhill in their drops (the lowest part of the curved handlebar on road bikes) because you pick up speed in that low, aerodynamic position, but it's the safest position for descending. Your weight is back and low, and you have good leverage to pull the brakes and brace your body in the proper position. The best way to get used to the feel of this simultaneous weight shift and brake pull is by practicing emergency stops, which exaggerates both motions but gives you an excellent feel for the physics of braking.

To pull an emergency stop, place both pedals parallel to the ground, lift your butt, and shift your weight way back behind the saddle. Extend your arms, and sink your weight low, dropping your torso toward the bike frame; then give your brakes a tight squeeze. Do this all in one smooth move, so it almost looks like you're trying to throw your bike forward and hurl your body back. Practice 5 or 6 times.

If you find these skills way too easy, make them harder. Start with your non-dominant foot on the pedal. Try to ride along a painted white line while scanning (in a parking lot or somewhere safe, of course!). Really home in on and perfect your braking so your stops are smooth and controlled.

THE BYBO RIDE

TERRAIN: Flat to gently undulating

WHAT TO DO	INTENSITY	HOW LONG
Warmup	ZONE 1–2	5 min
Steady effort	ZONE 2	5 min
Go hard	ZONE 3	3 min
Back down to easy	ZONE 1	2 min

Repeat that sequence (minus the warmup) 2 more times.

Finish at the pace of your choice going home.

TOTAL TIME: 40 min

Perform this workout 3 times this week.

NOTE: *If you're already riding for longer than 40 minutes, simply extend the beginning or end of your ride or add another interval sequence.*

TAKE-HOME: This workout is designed to help you gain confidence in basic bike handling as well as controlling your effort on the bike.

BYBO CORE WORKOUT
(SEE PAGE 24 FOR EXERCISE DIRECTIONS)

Do the moves one after another like a circuit. Then repeat.

- Plank
- Spider
- Bridge
- Dip

THE INSIDE RIDE

This workout incorporates a training style called cardioresistance (CR) training that blends cardio and strength training into the same workout. Researchers at Ithaca College found this high-energy mix builds fitness and sends strength soaring 25 percent in about half the time it usually takes to do both.

WHAT TO DO	INTENSITY	HOW LONG
Warmup	ZONE 1–2	5 min
Steady effort	ZONE 2	3 min
Increase resistance/effort	ZONE 3	3 min
Back off the effort	ZONE 2	2 min

Slow down and get off the bike.

Perform the BYBO Core Workout.

Get back on the bike and repeat the entire sequence (minus the warmup) once more.

Finish with 5–10 min of pedaling at the pace of your choice.

TOTAL TIME: 35 to 40 min

BYBO STRETCHES
(SEE PAGE 36 FOR STRETCH DIRECTIONS)

- Figure 4
- Stork
- Windshield Wiper

- Cobra
- Prayer Pose

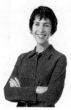

BIKE YOUR BUTT OFF! EATING PLAN: TUNE UP YOUR EATING HABITS

So you want to get fit, be fast, and feel fantastic? If you are reading this book, chances are that something about your eating habits needs to change. I would like you to spend Week 1 getting to know yourself and those habits a little better. Perhaps your speed, timing, or emotional eating could use some tweaking. Take a look at your plates, bowls, and glasses—you may need a bit of a "health-over."

Achieving self-accountability with food monitoring, logging, recording, whatever you want to call it and however you choose to do it, is the necessary first step. Too often people want to totally overhaul their eating but don't have a clue about what they are currently doing. How can we make changes if we don't know what we regularly do? How many times a day do you eat? Where do you eat? Are you a fast eater or a slow eater? We haven't even asked *what* you are eating because the speed, timing, and location are at least as important as the actual items and quantities you consume.

So how are you going to do this?

FOOD LOGS

Several kinds of logs are available, from the one provided on page 22 to online versions. But for the first week, I would really like you to use the one provided because we are asking you to record habits, and many of the online programs only have you record the foods you eat and the amounts.

Keep this food log for at least 3 days this week, and daily if possible. The purpose of this activity is for you to identify patterns and then pick the area(s) that you want to work on. In the first field you will note the date. In the second field, record what time you eat. The third field tracks where you eat (car, desk, kitchen counter). The fourth field is for the rate of eating (please time it; look at the clock when you start and again when you finish).

Then list the foods and beverages you consume. The more detail you provide, the more you'll get out of this. If you just write "sandwich," it is not nearly as revealing as "turkey and cheese on whole wheat with lettuce and tomato" or "meatball hero." So be specific. And that goes for the last field as well, which is for the amount. A glass could be a vat, and a plate could be a trough, and a handful could be a small jar. It is really helpful to use measuring cups and spoons to be very precise. Often when one is trying to lose weight, it is that pesky portion control that is the biggest barrier.

FOOD LOG ANALYSIS

Once you've accumulated food logs for at least 3 days, use the following guide to adjust your eating habits moving into the following week.

TIME OF DAY. Are your calories spread evenly throughout the day? Good. If not, I bet that you, like many people, are eating the majority of your food at night. Think about how you can redistribute those calories to have energy all day long, starting with your morning meal.

WHERE. Location, location, location—it's always essential. If you always eat in front of your computer and find yourself snacking soon after your meal, that should be a flag that you're not registering that you just ate because you're dis-tracted. Eating should be an event in and of itself—with a plate at a table. Take a hard look at where you eat and what effect it's having on your eating habits.

RATE. Winning the award for grab, gulp, and go? The "prize" is generally excess pounds. If it takes you less than 20 minutes to finish a meal, work on slowing down your eating to prevent overeating.

HOW MUCH. Your plate should be filled with reasonable portions. Three ounces of meat is about the size of a deck of cards or the palm of your hand. Grains, potatoes, pasta, and rice should be about the size of one tightly balled fist. A bagel should be the size of a hockey puck. The correct portions are probably a little smaller than you think they should be because we've been supersizing for more than a decade. Start cutting down to the right sizes. You won't miss the excess.

WEEK 1 *FOOD LOG*

Record everything you eat and drink (including amounts!) for at least 3 days this week, but 7 days if possible. Photocopy this page to use this log for the entire week.

DATE		TIME:	WHERE:	RATE:

FOOD/DRINK:

AMOUNT:

DATE		TIME:	WHERE:	RATE:

FOOD/DRINK:

AMOUNT:

DATE		TIME:	WHERE:	RATE:

FOOD/DRINK:

AMOUNT:

DATE		TIME:	WHERE:	RATE:

FOOD/DRINK:

AMOUNT:

DATE		TIME:	WHERE:	RATE:

FOOD/DRINK:

AMOUNT:

DATE		TIME:	WHERE:	RATE:

FOOD/DRINK:

AMOUNT:

DATE		TIME:	WHERE:	RATE:

FOOD/DRINK:

AMOUNT:

PLANK

Get down on the floor and balance on your toes and forearms. Keep your abs tight and your body in a straight line from heels to head. Work up to holding this position for 60 seconds.

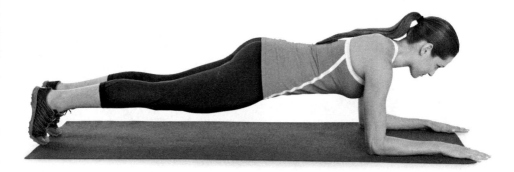

SPIDER

Holding light dumbbells (if you have them; if not, do the move without weights), get on all fours with your back straight, your hands directly beneath your shoulders so the weights are parallel with your body, and your knees directly beneath your hips. Raise your left arm straight out to the left side while simultaneously lifting your bent right leg out to the right side. Return to the starting position. Repeat on the opposite side. That's 1 rep. Do 12.

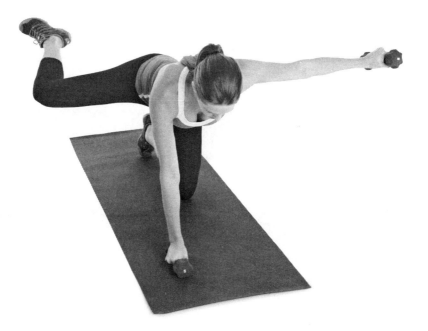

BRIDGE

Lie on your back with your knees bent, your feet flat on floor, and your arms at your sides, palms up. Contract your abs, press into your feet, and lift your butt and your lower and middle back off the floor. Then, straighten one leg and hold for a second. Lower your foot and then your body to floor. Repeat, alternating legs. Do 8 to 12 reps with each leg.

Make it easier: *Keep both feet on the floor at all times. Do 15 to 20 reps.*

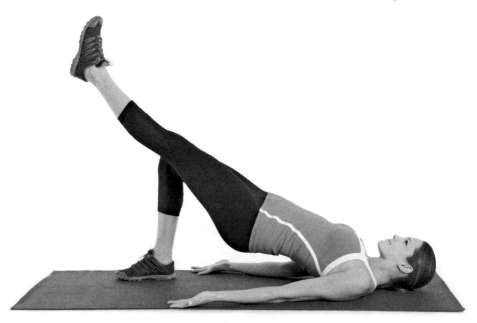

DIP

Sit on the edge of a chair (or a weight bench at the gym) with your hands grasping the seat on either side of your hips. Keep your knees bent and your feet flat on the floor. Scoot off the seat. Bend your elbows and lower your hips toward the floor until your upper arms are parallel with the floor. Straighten your arms and lift back to the starting position. Do 10 to 12 reps.

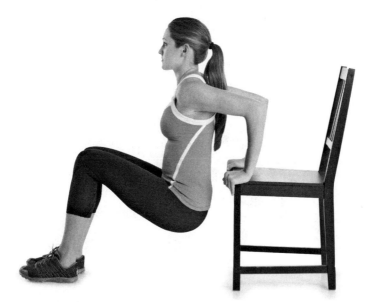

CRANK PLANK

Assume a side plank position, left arm extended, hand on the floor directly beneath your shoulder, feet stacked. Place your right hand behind your head, elbow pointing up. Keeping your hips stacked, slowly rotate your torso forward, bringing your right elbow toward the left arm. Rotate back to the starting position. Repeat for a full set of 10 reps. Then switch sides.

Make it easier: *Perform the move with the supporting arm bent, as shown here, so you're resting on your forearm.*

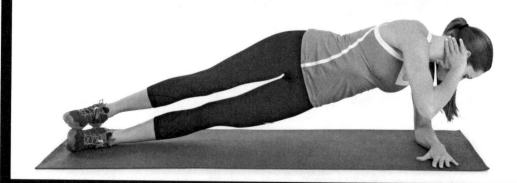

SPIDERMAN PUSHUP

Assume a pushup position with your arms extended, your palms flat beneath your shoulders, and your legs extended, feet flexed. Keep your abs tight. Bend your arms to lower your chest toward the floor. As you do, bend your right leg out to the side, bringing the right knee toward the right elbow. Pause, then return to the starting position. Switch sides. Repeat for a full set, alternating sides throughout. Do as many as you can.

Make it easier: *Perform the pushups from your knees, alternately lifting a knee off the floor as you lower your chest to the floor.*

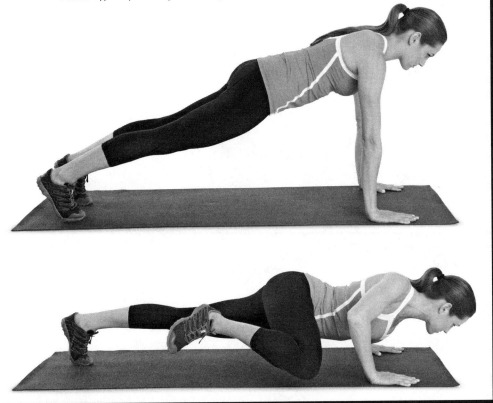

FIGURE 4 BRIDGE

Lie back on the floor with your knees bent to 90 degrees and your feet flat on the floor. Cross your right ankle over your left knee. Push into your left foot to raise your hips in the air so your body forms a straight line from your shoulders to your bent knee. Return to the starting position. Repeat for a full set of 10 reps. Then switch sides.

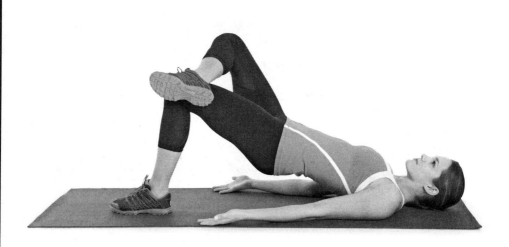

TIPPING BIRD

Stand tall with your arms out to the sides at shoulder height. Keeping your
right leg extended, lift your right foot behind you and balance on your left
leg. Slowly hinge forward from the hips, tipping your torso forward toward
the floor while extending your right leg straight behind you, foot flexed, until
your body forms a straight line from your head to your heel. Stop when
you're parallel with the floor. Return to the starting position. Switch sides.
Alternate for a set of 10 to each side.

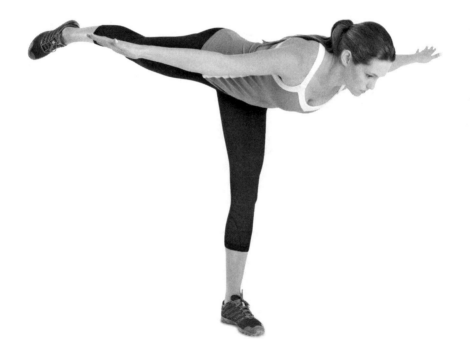

FOREARM PLANK WITH ARM RAISE

Get into the plank position (toes and forearms on the floor, body lifted). Your body should form a straight line. Brace your abs and carefully shift your weight to your right forearm. Extend your left arm in front of you and hold for 3 to 10 seconds. Slowly bring your arm back in. Repeat with the right arm. That's 1 rep. Do 5 to 10 reps.

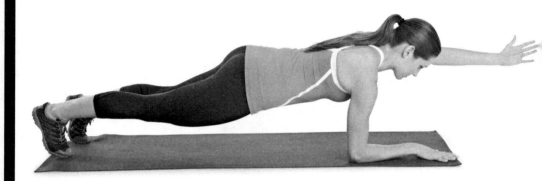

SIDE BRIDGE ABDUCTION

Lie on your left side with your elbow directly beneath your shoulder and your legs stacked. Brace your abs and lift your hips off the floor until you're balancing on your forearm and feet and your body forms a diagonal line. Lift your right leg by at least 6 inches. Lower and repeat. Complete 10 reps, then repeat on your right side. That's 1 set.

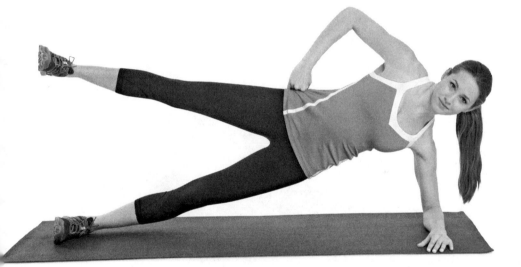

MOUNTAIN CLIMBERS

Start in a pushup position with a small towel under each foot (if you are on a carpeted floor, place a paper plate under each foot). Squeeze your shoulder blades together. Lengthen through the spine and pull your lower abs up toward the spine.

Without rocking or swaying the hips, slowly slide the left knee in toward your chest and slowly push it back out. Wait until the left leg is back in the starting position before you pull in the right knee.

Do 15 reps on each leg.

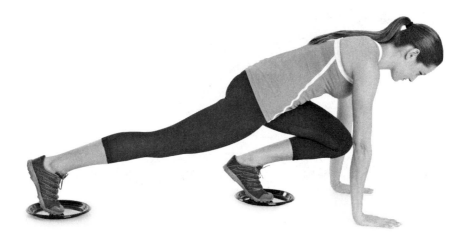

SCORPION

Lie facedown with your arms out to the sides, your shoulders flat on the floor. Lift your right leg off the floor and, twisting your torso, reach it across the back of your body as far as possible toward your left hand. Return to the starting position. Then repeat to the other side. Repeat for a full set of 10 reps to each side, alternating sides throughout.

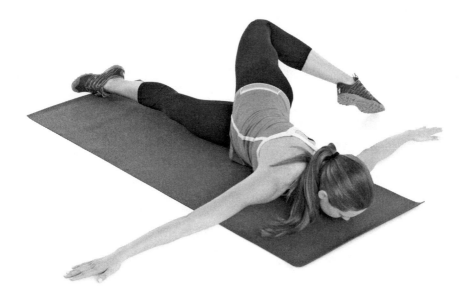

FIGURE 4

Sit up straight and tall in a chair, and cross one ankle over the opposite knee. Hinge forward until you feel a stretch throughout your hip. Hold for 30 seconds and then switch sides.

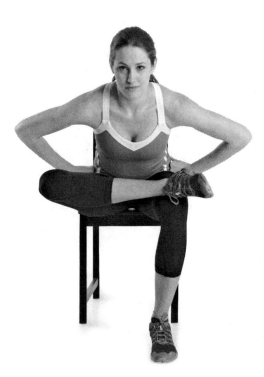

STORK

Stand with your feet together. Bend one leg and reach back and grasp that foot with the same-side hand. Keeping your knees in line, press your hips forward and gently pull your foot toward your rear to feel a stretch in your thigh. Hold for 30 seconds. Switch sides. (You can place the opposite hand on a wall or chair back for balance.)

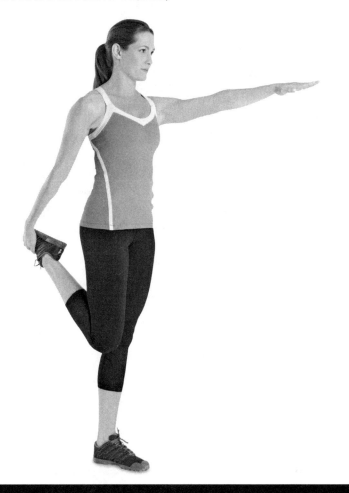

WINDSHIELD WIPER

Lie flat on your back with your arms outstretched and your hips and knees bent to 90 degrees. Allow your legs to fall as far as possible to one side while keeping your shoulders firmly on the floor. Pause for a second and then sweep your legs to the other side. Continue for 10 drops per side.

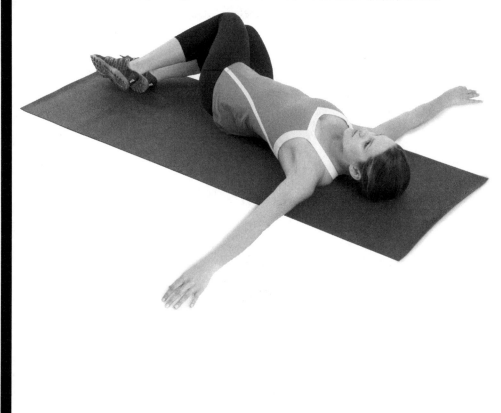

COBRA

Lie facedown with your feet together, toes pointed, and your hands on the floor palms down just in front of your shoulders. Lift your chin and gently extend your arms, lifting your upper body off the floor as far as comfortably possible. If you feel any strain in your back, alter the pose so that you keep your elbows bent and your forearms on the floor.

PRAYER POSE

From a kneeling position, sit back on your feet while stretching your arms as far as possible overhead. Press your hips back while dropping your torso toward the floor. Hold for 30 seconds.

CHAPTER 2

PUT THE
PEDAL
DOWN

NOW THAT YOU'VE BECOME acquainted with the basics of your bike, it's time to learn how to fully operate and enjoy it. For many new riders, that means getting to know the gears. Learning to shift into the right gear for the terrain you're on exponentially increases your comfort—and how fast and far you can ride.

While we're getting you comfortable, we'll also talk about key cycling comfort factors like saddle selection (as mentioned in Chapter 1, your seat is actually an interchangeable part), as well as about basic maintenance, like inflating tires, lubing your chain, and fixing a flat, which is good to know right out of the gate. On the weight-loss, eating side, we'll give you the tools you need to set weight-loss goals and, more important, achieve them. Let's get started.

GET YOURSELF IN GEAR

I can't count how many riders have asked, "Selene, what gear do you use?" when they start riding. My answer is always the same: "All of them. All the time." An essential skill for using your bike to improve your fitness and take you places—and to fully enjoying cycling as a lifelong sport—is understanding your gears and mastering gear selection.

Gears are designed to help you to pedal uphill, downhill, over flat land, and into a strong headwind without killing yourself, exhausting your muscles, or spinning your legs like a hamster on espresso. The most common gearing mistake new riders make is pedaling slowly in a high gear because they think cycling must feel like "work" every step of the way. Nothing could be further from the truth. Cycling is an aerobic activity, not resistance training. So, while you will feel your legs burn while you work up a particularly steep hill or if you're sprinting hard and fast, you should usually feel nothing but moderate pressure on your legs as you pedal. To achieve this, you need to shift early and often, especially if you live in a place that is undulating to hilly.

Here's how it works: As you saw in Chapter 1, most bikes have a series of gears, generally between 8 and 10, in the back on what is called a cassette. The biggest gear on the cassette (the one closest to your wheel) allows the easiest pedaling. The smallest gear is the hardest (good for slight declines). These gears are usually changed with the right-hand shift levers and allow you to make relatively small shifts. Think "right = rear" as a simple way to quickly remember which hand controls both your rear shifting and braking. So, if you're pedaling along and the road tips up a degree or two, you shift down to a lower gear to make the pedaling easier. Conversely, if the road tips down and you start pedaling too fast, you shift up to a higher gear.

In the front, attached to the crank arms that hold your pedals, you have chainrings. Most bikes have two or three chainrings. These gears are generally worked with your left-hand shift lever and are used to make more dramatic shifts. So if you're rolling along and the road or path pitches suddenly and steeply up, you shift from the big chainring into the smallest one to pedal more easily up the grade.

Shifting is as much an art as a science. But once you get it, you'll have it for good. Here are a few tips before we get to this week's Skill Drills and BYBO workouts.

PAY ATTENTION TO YOUR CADENCE. We'll talk in more detail about cadence (the rate at which you turn your pedals) in a later chapter. But for now, think "brisk." You don't want to be pushing down slowly on your pedals, but rather spinning your wheels in a brisk, comfortable rhythm. When you feel that brisk cadence start to slow, shift to an easier gear. When you feel it speed up too much, shift to a harder gear.

ANTICIPATE THE SHIFT. This is a golden rule for smooth shifting, and it requires you to use your eyes as much as your legs. When you see that the road is going to kick up, start shifting before you absolutely need to. Shifting when you're mashing down on your pedals trying to stay upright is a clunky affair. You want to be able to back off the force you're applying to your pedals to allow the chain to move smoothly. You can't do that under pressure.

KEEP A SMOOTH CHAINLINE. It's hard on your chain and gears to pedal along with your chain stretched at extreme angles. So if you're on your biggest chainring in the front as well as the biggest gear in the back, the pedaling may not be silky smooth as your chain tries to work under the tension that position generates. Generally, if you find yourself pedaling at those extremes for an extended time, you should shift onto another chainring (in this case to the smaller one) to smooth it out.

STAYING IN THE SADDLE

If you've gone from riding only sporadically (or never really riding) to clocking a lot of saddle time, there's a good chance your butt might hurt a bit at first. As mentioned in the previous chapter, padded cycling shorts will help a lot, but you may still have some tenderness over your sit bones.

That soreness should subside within the first 2 weeks. If it doesn't, consider changing your saddle. When you are perched on a properly fitting saddle, your weight should be supported by your sit bones on the flared rear of the saddle, without much pressure on your sensitive tissues. Your local bike shop sells both women's and men's saddles of every shape and size. They can help you find the one that suits you best.

One final note on butt comfort: Some riders may experience chafing, especially in damp weather, when the tender skin down under rubs against the inside of their shorts against the saddle. If that's a problem for you, you can head off unwanted hot spots by applying a gliding cream like Chamois Butt'r to the padding in your shorts.

BASIC MAINTENANCE

True story: I know a very smart, talented, and fit woman who barely took her $5,000 road bike outdoors to ride for the first 2 years she had it because

BIKE YOUR BUTT OFF! TOOL KIT

We'll talk all about the fun accessories that can improve your cycling life in later chapters, but for now, here are a few items that will keep you rolling.

TUBES. Inside your tires are inflatable tubes. Get yourself a few spares and carry one with you at all times. Tubes come in sizes to fit your wheels; check the outside of your tires for the correct dimensions. As mentioned on page 46, tubes come with one of two types of inflation valve, Presta or Schrader. Go with Presta, which are lighter.

TIRE LEVERS. Bike tires fit snugly on their rims. Tire levers help you pry them off when you need to fix a flat. They're light, cheap, and usually come in sets of three.

PUMP. You'll want two pumps—a nice floor pump for the garage and a minipump to carry with you. Floor pumps are quick and easy to use and have gauges that indicate the tube's air pressure. A minipump will easily fit in a pocket, so you can take it along in case you get a flat on the road.

LUBE. Pick up a bottle of chain lube to keep your chain running smooth and clean. There are many varieties to choose from, including wet, dry, and wax. Read the label to determine which type works best for your general riding conditions (rain, mud, dry, etc.).

she was afraid of having to fix a flat. Seems crazy until you realize that when you buy a bike, nobody really teaches you anything about maintaining or servicing it. I experienced this firsthand when I bought my first bike many moons ago.

Despite riding all through adolescence, I never once got a flat tire. It actually never occurred to me that you could get flat tires (I'm guessing my dad must've kept them pumped up for me). So, fresh out of school, I took a fistful of money I'd saved and bought a nice Specialized. On my maiden ride through one of the Philadelphia suburbs, I felt a squishy sensation in the rear. I stopped and looked back disbelievingly. The tire was completely flat. I didn't have a spare tube. I didn't have a single tool. And it wouldn't have done me any good even if I had, because I wouldn't have had a clue what to do. It was a very, very long walk home. I don't want this to happen to you.

As I emphasized last week, more than anything, I want you to be consistent and to make regular cycling a habit. That means eliminating as many roadblocks as possible. One such roadblock is basic bike maintenance and repair. Though your bike will likely work just fine 99 percent of the time, if you ride long enough, you eventually will encounter a "mechanical" (the term cyclists use for something that's gone wrong with the machine). Most commonly, that's a flat. One way to avoid flats is by keeping the tires properly inflated. Even if you never puncture your tubes, your tires eventually will go flat because air seeps through the tube's and tire's relatively porous rubber. Make it a habit to pump up your tires regularly, such as at the beginning of each week.

Road bike tires take considerably more pressure (in pounds per square inch [psi]) than mountain bike tires. Check the tire's sidewalls for the manufacturer's recommended pressure, and keep your tires inflated to that level. To pump up your tires, you first need to know what kind of valves the tubes have. There are two types: Presta and Schrader. Presta valves are skinny and have a locknut at the top that you unscrew and tap before applying the pump head to inflate it (then screw to tighten and keep the air in). Schrader valves are thicker and have a valve spring closure. Bike pumps generally adapt to work with either type of valve. Most cyclists opt for tubes with Presta valves. Keeping your tires properly inflated will help prevent what are known as pinch flats, when the tube gets squeezed between the rim and a hard surface like the edge of a pothole.

If you do happen to get a flat, keep your cool. It's an easy fix. Here's a step-by-step guide. I recommend practicing this at home to boost your confidence and so it feels automatic when you're out on the trail or road.

Remove the wheel. Your bike's wheels are easily removable—something many newbie riders don't know. Taking one or both wheels off makes it easy to slip a bike into a pickup bed, car trunk, or other tight space, as well as to fix a flat.

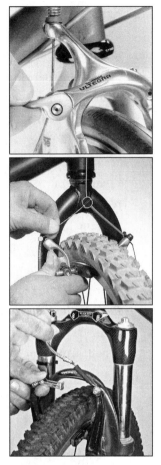

If the flat is in the back, create some slack in the chain by shifting into the smallest chainring and rear cog. Then open the brake.

On the front and rear wheels of road bikes, you'll see a little lever on the side of the braking mechanism. Lift that up, and you'll see the brake pads open wide from the rim, making room for your tire to pass through. If you don't see a lever, look for a button on the brake levers on the handlebars. Push that button. Mountain bikes often have linear or V-pull brakes; release those by squeezing the braking mechanism and lifting the brake cable out of its holder. Some bikes have cantilever brakes, with a cable centered above the tire; open those by releasing the cable from its holder near the brake pad on either side of the wheel. Disc brakes require no special steps; the disc simply slides out of the braking mechanism. This sounds complicated, I know. But trust me. It's not. Look at the pictures and see which one matches your bike. It will be obvious where the brake release is.

Next, open the quick release. Your wheel is attached to the bike frame by a skewer that sits in the hooks (called dropouts) on the bottom of your fork in the front and at the intersection of the seat stays and chain stays in the rear. That skewer is held tight with a locking mechanism called a quick release. Open the lever (it should be firmly cinched down) and hold the lever in place while turning the cap on the other side of the wheel a few times to loosen the release enough to remove the wheel.

Finally, remove the wheel. Front wheels slide right off. Rear wheels require more finesse. Pull the rear derailleur back and hold it there, so it and the chain are out of the way as you remove the wheel. Once the wheel is off, lean the bike over on its left side, so you don't get debris on your chain or bend the derailleur while you fix the flat.

Pull out the tube. Time to pull out your tire levers, spare tube, and pump (see page 45) and change the tube.

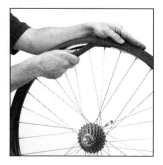

If the tire is not already completely flat, fully deflate it. For Presta valves, unscrew the top and press down to let the air out. For Schraders, stick an end of your tire lever into the valve and press the tip to release the remaining air. For Presta valves, once the air is out, remove the ring at the base of the valve to allow the tube to be removed.

Now use your levers to pull one side of the tire off the rim. Hold the wheel so that the valve is at the bottom, and wiggle the flat end of a lever between the rim and the tire. Wedge it under the edge (called the bead) of the tire. Pry the tire off the rim and hook the curved end of the lever to a nearby spoke. Now take another lever and do the same thing several inches away from the first lever. Repeat with the final lever. At this point, you should be able to move that entire side of the tire off the rim and pull out the tube. (If not, remove the first lever and pry off another spot until the tire comes loose.)

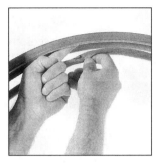

Check the tire. With the tube removed, check the inside of the tire for sharp objects. Sometimes you can see a thorn or sharp rock. Other times you may have to very carefully run your fingertips along the edges (the object could be glass, so use a light touch to avoid cutting yourself). It's possible that the offending item fell out when you pulled out the tube or that it punctured the tire and tube without getting lodged inside. But it's important to check so you don't get a second flat immediately after changing the first (been there; done that).

Replace tube and tire. Pull out your spare tube and pump it up just enough that it takes shape. Holding the wheel upright with the valve hole at the top, put the valve through the hole and tuck the tube into the tire and onto the rim with both hands, working your way down to the bottom of the wheel.

Now wriggle the tire back onto the rim. Fair warning: Tires fit tightly on the rims, so this can take some muscling. Starting at the valve, work the tire bead back into the rim using the palms of your hands. When you get to the bottom, it will become more difficult. Be sure that the valve is fully extended through the hole. If it feels impossibly tight, release some air from the tube. Then pull the final few inches of the tire back onto the rim.

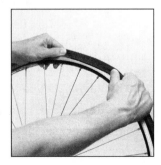

Pump, replace, and roll. Once the tire is back in place, add a little air and look between the rim's edge and the tire around the whole wheel to be sure the tube isn't sticking out anyplace (if it gets trapped under an edge, it can pop). Then finish inflating the tire. If you're using a minipump, you may not be able to inflate the tire to the same firmness you would with a floor pump. Just top it off when you get home.

Then put the wheel back on the bike, reversing what you did to take it off. For the rear wheel, pull back the derailleur and place the chain over the smallest cog. Then slide the skewer back through the dropouts. Tighten the quick release until you feel some resistance, and close it so the lever points up and aligns with the fork. It should be tight enough that it takes firm pressure to close the lever, but not so tight that you can't fully close it. Close the brake, and you're ready to roll.

After your tires, the most important bike part to maintain is your chain. Fortunately, it doesn't take much. You just need to keep it lubed. Lube keeps your chain and gears running smoothly by keeping dirt off the chain and away from your gears. To lube your chain, lean your bike against a wall and apply one drop of lube to each link as you slowly pedal backward. Once you've gone all the way around, continue pedaling for a few seconds to let the lube work its way into the chain. Then take a rag and gently press it against the chain as you pedal backward to wipe off the excess lube. It's a good idea to lube your chain after every few rides and always after riding in the rain, since water washes away the lube.

Finally, check your brakes regularly. It is important to keep them in good condition. Every time you squeeze your brakes, the pads wear a tiny bit. You don't want to let them wear all the way down, or you'll be rubbing metal on metal and be unable to stop. New pads have grooves to help channel water away from the rim so they get a better grip in wet conditions. When those grooves become worn nearly away, it's time to replace the pads. Your bike shop can do it in a snap.

SHED THE SPARE TIRE

So now that we've talked about your bicycle's spare tires, let's talk about yours. If you're turning these pages, there's a good chance you have a few pounds you'd like to lose. Our test panel volunteers ranged from very fit riders who wanted to firm up and get stronger to folks who'd let exercise fall by the wayside and wanted to reverse what had become an unwelcome amount of weight gain over the years. As mentioned in the introduction, cycling is the perfect vehicle for both ends of the spectrum because it burns hundreds of calories and is gentle on the joints. When you combine it with smart food choices, you will see a change on the scale. It's important, however, that you set realistic goals.

Over the years, the promise of how much weight you can lose on any given diet and exercise plan has been fairly exaggerated. We're not going to do that because it sets you up for long-term failure if you go into a program dreaming of dropping two sizes in 5 days and a week goes by and you're still wearing the same size.

So how much can you expect to lose? Realistically, half a pound to a pound a week—some weeks more, some less, depending on the food choices you make and how much you keep your body moving even when you're not on the bike. I know this sounds glacially slow to some people. But you lose weight the way you put it on, a bit at a time. Just as you didn't wake up one morning to find yourself 7 pounds heavier, you won't wake up one morning 7 pounds lighter. So do yourself a favor and put yourself in long-term-thinking mode right now. Time is going to pass no matter what you do. Days turn to weeks, which turn to months. Stay on the path, and a year from now you can be 20 or

30 (or more) pounds lighter. Or you can be the same. Or, like most Americans, you can be heavier. The choice is in your hands—and on your plate.

Leslie will help you make the transition to easy, healthy active eating. As you log your intake and make better choices, you can figure you'll probably be eating about 300 fewer calories a day (at least). To predict how much weight you'll lose over time based on how many calories you're cutting, check out the weight loss predictor at Pennington Biomedical Research Center (www.pbrc.edu/research-and-faculty/calculators/weight-loss-predictor). It's a good one, and it should help you stay on track to reach your goal weight.

Speaking of goal weights, I have one word of caution. Very often I ask people what their weight-loss goals are, and they spout out some crazy number from the time of their high school prom. If you weighed 115 pounds only once in your life and it was when you were 17, then that may not be a realistic goal. How do you know what's realistic? Medical professionals use the following formulas that factor in your height, gender, and frame size. Plug your numbers in here, and you'll have a weight you can likely attain—and live with.

STEP 1: BASELINE WEIGHT

The first step is determining your healthy base weight. Here's how you do it.

> **Women:** 100 pounds for the first 5 feet of height plus 5 pounds for each additional inch. For example, if you're 5 feet 6 inches tall, your ideal weight is 130 pounds (100 + 30).

> **Men:** 106 pounds of body weight for the first 5 feet of height plus 6 pounds for each additional inch. For example, if you're 5 feet 10 inches tall, your ideal weight is 166 pounds (106 + 60).

STEP 2: DETERMINE YOUR FRAME SIZE

Like bicycle frames, people come in all shapes and sizes. Your skeletal frame may be petite, or it may be large. That's why there's more than a 20-pound difference between the highest and lowest medically recommended weights for any given height. The best measurement of frame size is your wrist circumference in relation to your height. Measure your wrist with a tape measure and use the following chart to determine whether you are small, medium, or large boned.

WOMEN*

Height under 5'2"

Small = wrist less than 5.5"

Medium = wrist 5.5" to 5.75"

Large = wrist over 5.75"

Height 5'2" to 5'5"

Small = wrist less than 6"

Medium = wrist 6" to 6.25"

Large = wrist over 6.25"

Height over 5'5"

Small = wrist less than 6.25"

Medium = wrist 6.25" to 6.5"

Large = wrist over 6.5"

MEN

Height over 5'5"

Small = wrist 5.5" to 6.5"

Medium = wrist 6.5" to 7.5"

Large = wrist over 7.5"

ADJUST YOUR BASELINE: The baseline weight in the first step is based on a medium frame. For a small body frame, subtract 10 percent. For a large frame, add 10 percent.

Your number: _____

Women vary more by height and frame size than men do and therefore have more variation in this ratio.

WORKOUT: BE A SMOOTH OPERATOR

// SKILL DRILL: Run Your Gears

This week, get the hang of using your gears by running through them to see how each feels. Start with your front derailleur in the smaller of the two (or the middle of three) chainrings. Then, in a parking lot or on a safe, open stretch of road, start pedaling. As soon as you're rolling, shift up and down the cassette to get a feeling for upshifting and downshifting. Notice what happens with your pedaling speed and effort as you do. Repeat the exercise in your largest chainring, then again in your smallest.

Safety note: I don't want you to fall over in the parking lot or start weaving all over the road. So if you start to hit gears where you're having trouble keeping your pedaling smooth and the bike controlled, stop there. You've gotten the idea.

Finish this drill by picking your "go-to" gear. Yes, you should use all of your gears as conditions demand. But take a little time to find the one (or two) that allow you to pedal briskly and smoothly on flat ground. That should be your starting point.

CONSIDER A TRAINER

Turbo trainers, or simply "trainers," are triangular platforms that allow you to turn your outside bike into a stationary one that can be used anywhere in your home. They're perfect for when the weather turns too bad to get outdoors. You can plop them in front of the TV and watch your favorite sitcoms as you spin away. They're a great addition to help you stay in the saddle throughout and beyond the BYBO plan.

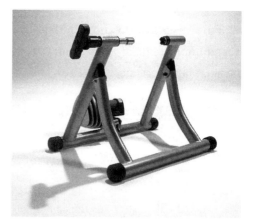

THE BYBO RIDE

TERRAIN: Flat to undulating, if possible

WHAT TO DO	INTENSITY	HOW LONG
Warmup	ZONE 1–2	5 min
Pedal briskly in your go-to gear*	ZONE 2	5 min
Pedal strong in a higher (harder) gear	ZONE 3	2 min
Pedal very fast in a lower (easier) gear	ZONE 3	1 min
Pedal briskly in your go-to gear*	ZONE 1–2	2 min

Repeat that sequence (minus the warmup) 2 more times.

Finish at the pace of your choice going home.

TOTAL TIME: 45–50 min

Perform this workout 3 times this week.

NOTE: *If you're already riding for longer than 40 minutes, simply extend the beginning or end of your ride or add another interval sequence.*

TAKE-HOME: This workout is designed to help you gain confidence in using your gears to control your pedaling cadence and effort. This will help you to complete longer rides with confidence. For more experienced riders, this is a good exercise in working muscles in a different way as you push against a bigger gear and spin rapidly in a small one.

Or the gear that matches your terrain.

THE INSIDE RIDE

Similar to last week, this workout incorporates cardioresistance training, which blends cardio and strength training into the same workout. This week, we'll mimic the outdoor ride and get you playing a bit more with resistance (which is like your outside bike's gear) and pedaling effort and speed.

WHAT TO DO	INTENSITY	HOW LONG
Warmup	ZONE 1–2	at least 5 min
Steady, brisk/moderate resistance	ZONE 2	5 min
Heavy resistance/effort	ZONE 3	2 min
Light resistance/fast pedaling	ZONE 3	1 min
Steady, brisk/moderate resistance	ZONE 1–2	2 min

Slow down and get off the bike.

Perform the BYBO Core Workout, repeating the circuit 2 times.

Get back on the bike and repeat the entire sequence (minus warmup) once more.

Finish with 5 min of pedaling at the pace of your choice.

TOTAL TIME: 45 min

BYBO CORE WORKOUT
(SEE PAGE 24 FOR EXERCISE DIRECTIONS)

Do the moves one after another like a circuit. Then repeat.

Plank

Spider

Bridge

Dip

BYBO STRETCHES
(SEE PAGE 36 FOR STRETCH DIRECTIONS)

- Figure 4
- Stork
- Windshield Wiper

- Cobra
- Prayer Pose

BIKE YOUR BUTT OFF! EATING PLAN: PUT THE PEDAL DOWN, PICK THE FORK UP!

I am all about finding balance between your intake and your output.

The intake is what and how much you eat and drink, and you did a lot of fact finding during your first week on the plan. So now we'll delve into energy expenditure and balance.

Your energy output comes from many sources, including your metabolism (how many calories you burn just being alive), your general activity, and your cycling and other exercise. The only way to get a firm, scientific number for your calorie output is to put you in a special chamber for a day, and we're not going to do that. So, we'll rely on some formulas instead. They're not exact—but they're pretty close.

1. First you need to know your basal metabolic rate (BMR), the number of calories your body burns at rest. Then you multiply your BMR by an activity factor, which will tell you how many calories you need to *maintain* your current weight.

2. The Harris-Benedict equations revised by Roza and Shizgal in 1984.

Men	BMR = 88.362 + (13.397 × weight in kg) + (4.799 × height in cm) − (5.677 × age in years)
Women	BMR = 447.593 + (9.247 × weight in kg) + (3.098 × height in cm) − (4.330 × age in years)

3. The following table enables calculation of the recommended daily calorie intake to maintain your current weight.

Then, factor in your activity level, using the following formulas.

Little to no exercise	Daily calories needed = BMR × 1.2
Light exercise (1–3 days per week)	Daily calories needed = BMR × 1.375
Moderate exercise (3–5 days per week)	Daily calories needed = BMR × 1.55
Heavy exercise (6–7 days per week)	Daily calories needed = BMR × 1.725
Very heavy exercise (twice per day, extra-heavy workouts)	Daily calories needed = BMR × 1.9

Since your goal is likely to lose weight rather than maintain, you would take the number you get from multiplying your BMR by the appropriate activity level and subtract 250 to 300 calories, which would yield a weekly weight loss (according to your amount of body fat) of about $1/2$ to $3/4$ pound per week. I don't want you to cut too many calories or you won't have the energy to ride, and Selene will kill me!

In addition to your BMR, you also burn calories through non-exercise activity thermogenesis (NEAT). In other words, sit less and fidget or move more to burn additional calories daily.

Last but not least, we add in the thermic effect of feeding (TEF). Your body has to burn calories to digest the food you eat, but before you get too excited, the calories burned are few, and this does not mean you should eat 25 times a day. Recent studies suggest that eating three times a day is enough to get the TEF benefit. So even though some plans suggest eating six times a day, I think this is too many, and it often results in excessive calorie intake.

So now that we have your daily output, let's calculate what you should be taking in to hit your weight loss goals.

(Your BMR × activity factor) – (250 to 300 calories) =

_____ YOUR DAILY CALORIES FOR WEIGHT LOSS

TRACKING YOUR FUEL INTAKE

This week, I would like you to keep track of the calories you consume. This is mostly an exercise in fact finding. You may not be able to find the calorie counts for everything you eat, but you will see them on packaged foods, and restaurants often post calories as well. Remember, when you look at packaged foods, the most important lines are the top two: serving size and number of servings per container. The nutrition facts, including calories, are based on *one* serving, which in some cases is the whole container, bottle, or bag, but not always!

In addition, there are several online programs that will help you find the calorie counts of common foods:

- CalorieKing:
  www.calorieking.com

- MyFitnessPal:
  www.myfitnesspal.com

- Livestrong:
  www.livestrong.com

- MyFood-a-Pedia:
  apps.usa.gov/myfood-
  a-pedia.shtml

So either flip the package and read the label or do a search, but know the number of calories you are putting into your mouth.

Now, back to the kitchen and your eating environment. If your goal is to

(continued on page 62)

WEEK 2 *FOOD LOG*

This week, make sure you are counting calories in addition to recording everything you eat and drink. As before, you can make additional photocopies of this page to use for the whole week.

Food logging is a powerful weight-loss tool, so feel free to use copies of this page to log your daily food and drink for the duration of the program.

DATE	TIME:	WHERE:	RATE:
FOOD/DRINK:			
AMOUNT:			TOTAL CALORIES:

DATE	TIME:	WHERE:	RATE:
FOOD/DRINK:			
AMOUNT:			TOTAL CALORIES:

DATE	TIME:	WHERE:	RATE:
FOOD/DRINK:			
AMOUNT:			TOTAL CALORIES:

DATE	TIME:	WHERE:	RATE:

FOOD/DRINK:

AMOUNT: | TOTAL CALORIES:

DATE	TIME:	WHERE:	RATE:

FOOD/DRINK:

AMOUNT: | TOTAL CALORIES:

DATE	TIME:	WHERE:	RATE:

FOOD/DRINK:

AMOUNT: | TOTAL CALORIES:

DATE	TIME:	WHERE:	RATE:

FOOD/DRINK:

AMOUNT: | TOTAL CALORIES:

WEEK 2

have a leaner, fitter you, you need to create an eating environment that is conducive to success. Out of house, out of mouth. If the tempting foods are around, you know very well what you are going to choose, so get a garbage bag and clean out the cabinets, desk drawers, car, refrigerator, and freezer. This is an exercise in not just taking away, but also adding in. What should you stock?

Time to create your own Tour de Store! Here is a shopping list to get you started.

1. A variety of colorful fruits and 100 percent fruit juices
2. A variety of vibrantly colored vegetables, including dark-green vegetables, starchy vegetables, red-orange vegetables, beans, and peas
3. Whole, enriched, and fiber-rich grain-based foods
4. Low-fat and fat-free milk, cheese, and yogurt
5. Lean meats, poultry, fish, eggs, nuts, and seeds

The list at right is from the Nutrient Rich Foods Coalition (www.nutrient richfoods.org). Don't feel that you have to buy everything on this list. It is a starting point. Take a look at the list, circle the foods you like and will eat (and know how to cook) and start with those, in the quantity that works for you. If you are buying for one, it doesn't really make sense to buy a family-size bag of apples. Buy only what you need.

In general, try to keep these guidelines in mind when you shop—whether for meal ingredients or for snacks. Strive for more foods from the Best Bets category and fewer from the To Watch category.

PROTEIN	GRAINS	FRUITS/VEGETABLES
Beef	Rice	All fresh fruits
Chicken	Pasta	Canned fruits in juice
Seafood	Potatoes	Salads
Turkey	Bread	Steamed vegetables
Pork	Cereal	Grilled vegetables
Eggs/egg whites	Grits	Roasted vegetables
Cheese	Oatmeal	Stir-fried vegetables
Cottage cheese	Pita	Beans
Greek or low-fat yogurt	Wraps	Edamame
Low-fat milk		Baked white or sweet potatoes
Low-fat soy milk		Frozen fruit bars

// TO WATCH (HIGHER IN CALORIES, FAT, OR BOTH)

PROTEIN	GRAINS/SWEETS	FRUITS/VEGETABLES
Fried meats	Biscuits	Dried fruits (in large amounts)
Chicken nuggets	Cookies/pies/pastries	French fries
Salami	Doughnuts	Onion rings
Bologna	Sweetened cereals	Juice drinks/fruit punch
Hot dogs	Corn chips	Potato chips
Pepperoni	Soda	
Pizzas	Sweet tea	
	Ice cream	
	Candy	

Secrets of Their Success

BECKY ROUSH, 35

WEIGHT LOST:
3½ pounds,
plus 1 inch off
her waist

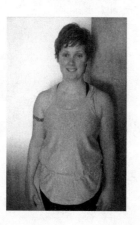

Becky had been riding on and off—mostly off—since 2007. In 2012, she decided she wanted to start riding on a regular basis, including riding her bike to work at least one day a week. She also signed up for a couple of longer charity rides. She came to the BYBO plan hoping it would jump-start a regular riding habit and improve her bike-handling and riding skills. Getting a bit stronger and fitter would be a bonus.

She accomplished all the above. She began commuting the 8 to 10 miles (depending on which route she chose) to her job in Pittsburgh more regularly. She also did more riding in general, hitting the city trails with her husband and signing up for an MS 150 charity ride to be held in the spring following the BYBO program. She worked hard to soak in the BYBO lessons and reaped the rewards quickly. In just a few short weeks of following the BYBO plan, she found herself kicking her husband's butt on their trail outings and enjoying improvements in nearly every aspect of her riding.

"The lesson plans are very well presented and organized, which helped with steady improvement. I have definitely become stronger and I have made my pedaling more efficient. I also am better at carrying speed through tight corners, which makes a big difference getting places and increases my confidence on taking less tight corners with some speed," she says. "I would like to take time in the near future to revisit some of the lessons—especially the one on paying attention to your cadence. I can see myself (and my husband) doing them again together in the near future."

Becky is also committed to learning to layer her clothing so she can commute year-round. "I ordered a rain jacket, have full-finger gloves, and am picking up some shoe covers," she told us, adding, "I like to drink beer, so I need to keep riding even when it's cold!"

Speaking of beer, Becky made some positive changes to her diet, especially during the week, nixing alcohol until the weekends and also using the weekends to cook good, healthy foods to eat during the week, when she's too busy with work and school to do much meal prep. The final touches of cleaning up her diet included swapping sugary cider for unsweetened tea and having a little snack after her hard rides to prevent her from feeling ravenous (and overeating) later in the day.

Unfortunately, Becky also experienced her first bike wreck during one of her commutes. However, she kept her head, maneuvered the best she could to avoid a direct collision, and minimized the damage. "A car stopped quickly in front of me as I was avoiding potholes and couldn't stop in time. I tried to cut over between it and the parked cars, but my pannier caught the bumper. He was very nice, the bike is okay, and so am I, barring a few spectacular bruises. I am more careful now," she says.

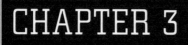

CHAPTER 3

ENJOY
THE
RIDE

ASK CYCLISTS WHAT THEY love most about the sport, and you'll think you were talking to a group of aspiring pilots.

"It feels like flying."

"The freedom."

"The views."

When was the last time you felt like you were flying when you were exercising? Yeah, I thought so. In my mind, that's what sets cycling apart from other forms of physical activity. Most of the people I know who ride their bikes ride them not to get exercise, but because of how wonderful it makes them feel. They ride because there's nowhere else they can feel like a kid, free and unfettered, out exploring the world on their own two wheels. Because there's nowhere else where 10 or 15 minutes of suffering can be rewarded with stunning views and soaring descents. There's simply nothing else like it.

The entire purpose of this book, of course, is to help you develop the skills and fitness to take the leap from the nest and really fly on your bike, and see weight-loss goals come to life in the process. To that end, this week we'll continue to work on skills like cornering that can be a bit intimidating but increase your enjoyment exponentially once you get good at them. We'll also discuss music (a must when you're stuck inside) and start getting you psyched up (and prepared) to start doing long rides.

GO WITH THE FLOW

The fastest way from point A to point B may be a straight line, but rarely is it the most fun. The best trips by bike are filled with twists and turns and glorious sweeping curves. So it's best to know how to steer, which on a bike is a little different from turning the wheel on a car.

You actually steer your bike more with your body than you do with your handlebars, because turning and cornering are mostly about leaning the bike in the direction you want to go. You can see this at work without even getting on your bike. Simply walk your bike along a straight line, then, holding onto just the saddle, tip the bike in one direction and see what happens—it turns. Flat, easy turns require little more than a slight turn of the bars and a lean with both body and bike. As the turns become steeper (such as going down a hill), however, good cornering takes a bit more finesse.

To take sharp corners like a pro, you use a cool little maneuver called countersteering, which is to say you steer a little bit in the direction you don't want to go before launching the bike in the desired direction. Sounds complicated, but once you try it you'll see how easy it really is. To get the picture, imagine you're making a quick, sharp right-hand turn. As you approach the corner, you turn ever so slightly to the left. Almost instantaneously, you'll lean right to maintain balance. As you lean right, you then turn to the right and sweep around the bend.

Here are a few tips that will help smooth those turns and corners.

GET LOW. You'll feel more secure steering through sharp turns if you keep your center of gravity low. That means using the drops (the lowest part of your curvy bars on a traditional road bike) on a road bike or simply bending your elbows and dipping your torso a bit on a flat-handlebarred bike.

RIDE LOOSE. Since you're cornering with your whole body, you need your hips, feet, hands, and torso free to move. That means keeping loose! If you tense up, your arms will straighten, and you'll end up fighting your bike through the turn. As you approach a turn, consciously relax your hands and arms so you have a firm, but not white-knuckle tight, grip on the bars and your upper body feels loose. Your elbows should be bent.

SCRUB SPEED AHEAD OF THE CURVE. Hitting the brakes makes your bike sit up and straighten out. That's not the position you want to be in when you are turning. You want to get most, if not all, of your braking out of the way before you get to your corner so you can coast through the turn with minimal braking, if any. To do this, feather your brakes (i.e., squeeze the levers just enough to caress the rims) as you approach the turn. You should barely feel your weight going into your bars. If your weight shifts forward, you're squeezing too hard. Then let go once you're in the turn, feathering again only if necessary.

PRESS INTO YOUR PEDAL. For sharp turns, you want to keep your wheels planted firmly on the ground (and avoid skidding) by weighting your wheels. Extend your outside leg and push very heavily into the pedal as you lightly press down on the handlebar with your inside hand. This will help you maintain traction as you sweep through the curve.

LOOK WHERE YOU WANT TO GO. Your bike follows your eyes, much as your body follows your eyes. So look through the corner to where you want to go. Pay attention to what some pros call your third eye (your navel). That, too, should be "looking" (pointed) in the direction you want to go, as it ensures your hips and torso are carrying you through the turn. Remember, you're steering with your full body. So point your eyes and chin and shoulders in the direction you want to go, and the rest will follow.

TAKE THE LONG WAY

I remember when I first started riding as a teen, I was thrilled about the world of possibilities that suddenly sprawled out beneath my wheels. I didn't have to rely on my parents to drive me around. I could hop aboard my bike and visit my friend Deanna (8 miles, mostly uphill there; downhill home). I could go see Sheila (a mere 3 miles through town). I could even go to the lake (10 miles, very hilly but very beautiful). When I rediscovered riding as an adult, I rediscovered that thrill. Sure, I can drive now. But when my friends invited me to ride 20 miles to Uptown Espresso Bar in Kutztown, Pennsylvania, or 45 out to Hawk Mountain, my heart would leap a little. Going by bike turns any trip into a fun little adventure.

How do you know when you're ready to take a longer trip? If you've pedaled comfortably for 30 to 60 minutes, from a *fitness* standpoint you're ready to tackle a challenge of, say, $1^1/_2$ to 2 hours. You may be less ready depending on your comfort level regarding skills, bike handling, and riding with traffic. All of this will come with more practice. I'm confident that by the end of this program, you'll be ready to tackle nearly any cycling adventure. But early on, you can keep yourself in your comfort zone by asking your riding friends (or yourself if you're planning a solo venture) a few quick questions.

HOW ARE THE ROADS? Will the trip be on quiet country roads or busier main arteries? If the latter, do they have a wide shoulder? You want your first big outings to be as enjoyable as possible. Sticking to quieter roads until you're comfortable on busier throughways will help.

WHAT IS THE TERRAIN? You never quite appreciate the grade of even a small hill until you do it by bike. What looks like "nothing" behind the wheel of your car will feel like "something" beneath the wheels of your bike. This is not a bad thing. Hills make you strong. But if you're not conditioned for them, they can tire you out much more quickly than flat roads.

HOW FAR? HOW FAST? Speed and duration have sort of an inverse relationship for many new riders, who can go a good distance or pedal very fast, but still don't have the muscular endurance (more on that later) to put them together. So if you're going with others you haven't yet ridden with, it's reasonable to ask how fast the group will move. No matter if you're going alone or with others, you should have a good idea of how far the trip will be. Twenty miles (round-trip) is a good beginning target if you're taking your own sweet time.

Though you can certainly tackle some longer trips without any special gear, a few additions to your cycling closet can make it more comfortable to spend a couple of hours in the saddle.

JERSEY. Do you need a special shirt to ride your bike? No. Will you love one once you own one? Yes. Cycling jerseys come equipped with special features

THESE SHOES ARE MADE FOR RIDING

Now is also a good time to start thinking about clipless pedals. The name "clipless," which is a bit of a misnomer, refers to the fact that these pedals don't have toe straps and cages (which used to be commonplace for securing the rider's foot to the pedal), but instead actually clip to the shoes via a cleat on the soles. If you're really enjoying cycling for fitness and recreation, clipless pedals can help take your riding to the next level by providing optimum pedaling comfort and efficiency.

The special cycling shoes you use with clipless pedals not only firmly attach to the pedal, they also have stiff soles that ensure all the energy from your pedaling transfers into propelling you down the road. They also help keep your feet from fatiguing on long rides. Learning to ride clipless takes a little time and practice, of course. It is also a bit of a financial investment to purchase the special cycling shoe–pedal combination. It may not be something you're ready for at this moment, but it's definitely worth thinking about and investigating as you continue along the road to becoming a cyclist.

First you need to decide which clipless pedal system is right for you. Most pedal manufacturers make clipless pedals for both road and mountain bikes. Mountain shoes have rugged soles that are easier to hike unridable sections in. Road shoes are smooth soled. Mountain bike pedals tend to have a smaller cleat (the part that attaches to your shoe) but a larger pedal platform and are designed to be easy to use even in dirty or muddy conditions. Road pedals often have larger cleats to provide a that raise the enjoyment factor on any ride. For one, they're specially tailored for the job at hand—that is, they are cut so they hug your body closely without flapping in the breeze, and they're longer in the back and shorter in the front, so they don't scrunch up around your belly and ride up, exposing your back when you're perched forward in the cycling position. They

greater surface area to distribute the pedal pressure and keep your feet comfortable on long rides. The other distinguishing factor among pedals is the amount of "float" they have, or how much side-to-side movement they allow. Some pedal systems lock your foot in place very tightly, while others allow more play. Generally a little play is better for your knees. Your bike shop salesperson can help you find the pedal system that is best for your riding needs.

Once you've picked your pedals, it's time to learn the art of clipping in and out. To get "clipped," you step onto the pedal, applying pressure toe to heel until you feel the cleat and pedal engage (you'll also hear a "click"). To unclip, you turn your heel out while pulling up. It's a fairly simple process, but I won't lie, you're bound to tip over once or twice because you don't clip out in time when coming to a stop. A little practice can help you avoid the ever-embarrassing stop-sign topple.

To start, place your bike next to a wall or fixed object that you can easily prop yourself against while sitting on the saddle. Sit on the bike and lean against the wall with your right arm, leaving the right foot unclipped and resting on the pedal platform. With the left pedal in the down (six o'clock) position, practice clipping and unclipping with your left foot. Repeat until it comes easily. Flip the bike around and practice on the other side.

When you're ready, find a flat, wide-open space (grassy fields work well) to practice on the fly. Ride for 30 seconds or so, then slowly come to a stop while clipping out. Keep practicing. As you become more comfortable, try stopping and clipping out more quickly. The more you practice, the more naturally it will come out on the open road.

have a front zipper to help you cool down quickly when the going gets hot and are generally constructed with sweat-wicking synthetic materials. Best of all, they have pockets in the back, usually two or three, for stashing keys, cash, fig bars, a light jacket, and anything else you might need for your trip.

COMPUTER. It's very fun (and satisfying) to know how far you've ridden on any given outing. A cycling computer can tell you that and much, much more. Basic computers include a small digital screen that affixes to your handlebar and communicates with a sensor fixed to your front wheel. Together they register how fast you're going, how far you've traveled, your maximum speed, your average speed, and how long you've been riding (also see the discussion of GPS on page 108).

GLOVES. Padded cycling gloves help absorb the bumps and vibration from your wheels on the road to keep your hands from getting sore or numb. They also help prevent your hands from slipping on the bars when it's hot (and you're sweaty) or when it's drizzly. Plus, if you do happen to take a spill, they protect your hands from scrapes and abrasions.

SUNGLASSES. Sports-specific sunglasses will protect your peepers not only from the sun's harmful UV rays, but also from road debris, bugs, and other potential projectiles that can find your eyes at the most inopportune times. Cycling shades also generally come with interchangeable lenses, so you can use light lenses for overcast days and darker ones when the sun's burning bright.

LET THE MUSIC PLAY

Cycling is such a pleasure in and of itself that I don't advocate riding with an iPod. It's far better (and, let's face it, safer) to soak in the sights and sounds uninterrupted as you ride. That said, if you ride indoors, music is a must. I also really love a good soundtrack when I'm performing intervals at the local park, which is far removed from traffic and a place where I feel very safe being a little tuned out. (Even when I'm zipping around this safe open space, I still keep one ear open to my surroundings by using an earbud from One-Good Earphones. It's an earphone that channels the stereo sound from your iPod into a single earbud.)

Music is a scientifically proven performance enhancer. One recent comprehensive research review reported in detail how music lowers your perceived effort (how hard you feel like you're working), boosts your endurance, and pleasantly distracts your mind from pain and fatigue, all of which allows you to push harder and longer than you would in complete silence.

One of my favorite times to use music is actually *before* I ride, when I'm sitting at my desk stuck in a pool of inertia, knowing that I *should* ride and that I'll feel great once I get changed and get on my bike, but, well, you know . . . getting moving is the hardest part. At those moments, cuing up a little motivation music (and it can be anything from Nelly to Nine Inch Nails) helps put me in motion. The right music also can keep you in motion, as research finds that we tend to sync up with the beat of whatever is playing, which of course is why aerobics instructors play such high-energy tunes.

You can make your own playlist to match every workout by knowing the typical beats per minute (bpm) of the music you like. The following chart is a good guide. If you want to get more precise, you can download a free music analyzer app like the MixMeister BPM Analyzer, which rates the bpm of the songs in your library.

FOR THIS TYPE OF RIDING	IDEAL BPM	BEST GENRE
Recovery	~100–110	Country/hip-hop
Intervals	~160+	Heavy metal
Tempo	~140–150	Techno/rock
Endurance	~120–130	Pop/alternative

WORKOUT: TURN THE CORNER

// **SKILL DRILL:** Taking Turns

Michael Phelps didn't spend 15 years practicing kicking drills in the pool because he didn't know how to kick. He did it so that when he got into the heat of competition he didn't have to think about executing the perfect flutter—it was automatic. The same applies for turning and cornering. You want to make the right motions automatic, so there's no thinking required when you approach the real thing. In a parking lot, empty industrial park, or other open, car-free space, perform the following moves.

TURNS AND S-TURNS. First practice a series (five or six) of right-hand turns with varying degrees of steepness. Then repeat to the left. Finish by stringing together four or five slalom turns to each side, which means going back and forth (making swooping turns to each side).

CIRCLES. Put your bike in a low gear and ride in slow left-hand circles, gradually picking up speed and bringing the circle tighter and tighter, staying in control the entire time. With practice, you should be able to make those circles smaller and smaller. Practice in both directions. It's not uncommon for riders to find it easier to turn in one direction than the other.

FIGURE EIGHTS. Finally, move on to figure eights, which are perfect practice for real-life riding because you have to change directions quickly to maintain control. This is where you should really feel countersteering at work.

THE BYBO RIDE

TERRAIN: Flat to undulating

WHAT TO DO	INTENSITY	HOW LONG
Warmup	ZONE 1–2	~5 min
Pedal briskly; take turns smoothly	ZONE 2	15 min
Increase effort; pedal out of any corners and turns, concentrating on maintaining your effort with minimal coasting	ZONE 2–3*	10 min
Back to brisk; keep corners and turns smooth	ZONE 2	15 min

Finish at the pace of your choice going home.

TOTAL TIME: ~45–50 min

Perform this workout 3 times this week.

NOTE: *If you're already riding for longer than 45 minutes, simply extend the beginning or end of your ride or add another interval sequence.*

TAKE-HOME: This workout brings together all the skills you've worked on thus far, while keeping you pedaling at a smooth and steady pace. The ride should start to feel seamless by the final session.

*This effort should feel like it's on the breaking point between aerobic and hard.

THE INSIDE RIDE

Similar to last week, this workout incorporates cardioresistance training, which blends cardio and strength training into the same workout. Once again, we'll mimic the outdoor ride and concentrate on smooth, steady pedaling.

WHAT TO DO	INTENSITY	HOW LONG
Warmup	ZONE 1–2	~2–3 min
Steady, brisk, moderate resistance	ZONE 2	10 min
Increase effort (> resistance and/or faster pedaling; stay smooth)	ZONE 2–3*	5 min
Smoothly ease off the effort	ZONE 2 to 1	2–3 min

Perform the BYBO Core Workout.

Get back on the bike and repeat the entire sequence (minus the warmup) once more (but perform just one circuit of the Core Workout this time).

Finish with some easy stretching.

TOTAL TIME: 45–50 min

This effort should feel like it's on the breaking point between aerobic and hard.

WORKOUT LOG

Please log your workouts for the week.

WEEK 3				
BYBO Rides (including pleasure cruise) and Core Workouts	Date: Notes:	Date: Notes:	Date: Notes:	Date: Notes:
Cross-training and/or rest	Date: Activity: Duration:	Date: Activity: Duration:	Date: Activity: Duration:	Date: Activity: Duration:

ANY OBSTACLES? _____

ACCOMPLISHMENTS? _____

OTHER NOTES: _____

BYBO CORE WORKOUT
(SEE PAGE 24 FOR EXERCISE DIRECTIONS)

Do the moves one after another like a circuit. Then repeat.

Plank   Bridge

Spider   Dip

BYBO STRETCHES
(SEE PAGE 36 FOR STRETCH DIRECTIONS)

Figure 4   Cobra

Stork   Prayer Pose

Windshield Wiper

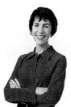

LESLIE'S LESSONS

BIKE YOUR BUTT OFF! EATING PLAN: CONDUCT AN INTERNAL INVESTIGATION

Let's pull out those food logs and do a little investigation. What are the troubling times of day when your willpower heads south and too much food heads north to your mouth? Where are you eating the most? At the table? Or standing at the sink? How quickly are you eating?

Making meaningful changes in your food habits typically takes 12 weeks, but modifying those habits is a step-by-step process that happens on every day of the weight-loss journey. A huge part of that journey is setting the stage for success in every way possible. I often find that when my clients are in action mode, they focus on changing what's on the plate, but they tune out everything else. In order to be successful with weight loss, brain and body need to be on the same page. To do this, you need to create a healthy environment for eating success. Here are the suggestions for Week 3.

ESTABLISH NO-EATING ZONES. Think of how many establishments are now smoke-free. Similarly, you need to have food-free zones, banning yourself from eating in certain places where you can't fully focus on what you're consuming. Why? Being able to focus on what you are eating increases the likelihood that you pay attention to hunger and fullness. Identify some of these places this week: In the car? In the bathroom? While you are at your computer or in front of the TV? You decide which spaces you can eliminate as eating zones and also identify what areas will be your eating spaces.

CHOOSE MEAL TIMES. Although there is no single "right" number of meals to consume daily, there are a lot of wrong ones. On the one hand, eating once a day is not going to cut it because you will have long periods of time without food, which means you won't have enough energy to ride. On the other hand, there is no need to eat every hour either. So many diet plans suggest eating six small meals a day—I do not. The problem is that if you are eating all the time, how will you ever know if you are hungry or not? And as far as boosting the metabolism, recent studies have shown that eating three times a day has the same effect on the metabolic rate as eating six times, whereas eating six times a day can increase the chance that you are overconsuming calories. So choose how many meals you would like each day and the approximate times you would like to have them.

In terms of spacing out your meals, the goal is to eat enough at a meal that you could go 4 to 5 hours until you eat again. This is another reason for keeping food logs—so you can see how long you can go between meals. I think you'll find that the more satisfying the meal, the longer you can go. If you feel the need to eat every 2 hours, perhaps you should consolidate two of those eating occasions into one larger, more satisfying meal; you might discover that 4 hours have passed before you feel the need to eat again.

FORGO GRAZING. Once you've established your mealtimes, stick with them and cease snacking all day. What's wrong with grazing? It's mindless. Most people graze while standing up, walking, watching TV, etc. And what are you grazing on? Carrots? Hah! More likely it is savory snacks, sweets, or cereal out of the box. When eating hand to mouth, no utensils required, often the food is practically inhaled.

If you are a grazer, all those little bits of food add up, and truthfully, you probably never feel full even though your mouth is working overtime. So how to be an eater versus a grazer? Put your food on a plate or in a bowl. Get your butt in the chair and a utensil in your hand. This way you know what and how much you are eating.

RANK HUNGER VERSUS APPETITE. What makes you eat? Is it always in response to hunger? I don't think so. We eat when we're happy, sad, bored, or mad. We eat to celebrate, for comfort, and just for something to do. However, if you want to see a change on the scale and in your clothes, you are going to want to get to the point where the majority of eating occasions occur in response to hunger. So this week you are going to identify what happens when you eat, and you will mark your food log accordingly. Hunger is an internal cue of the body's need for food—your stomach growls, you might feel slightly headachy, sometimes even a little light-headed. Let's contrast this with appetite—external cues—the desire for food. For example, you've just eaten lunch, but someone brings in brownies. You aren't really hungry, but you have one (or five) because they look good. The problem with eating according to appetite is that we may have already consumed our allotted calories, but we keep eating because the food looks good, smells good, and is available!

WEEK 3 FOOD LOG

In the food log for this week, I would like you to keep track as follows:

Column 1: Date.

Column 2: Time you are eating.

Column 3: Indicate whether the eating occasion is a meal or snack. List every eating occasion separately so that you can see how many unique times you are eating every day.

Column 4: List what you eat and/or drink.

Column 5: Indicate whether you are eating out of hunger (H) or because of appetite (A). This could be because the food was there, someone else was eating, it smelled good, etc.

Column 6: For each meal or snack, rate your hunger *before* you eat on a scale of 1 to 5 (1 = not hungry at all; 5 = *starved*).

Column 7: For each meal/snack you eat, rate your fullness *after* eating on a scale of 1 to 5 (1 = still hungry; 5 = *stuffed*).

Use the following log to further refine the parameters of your eating, snacking, and meal timing. You can photocopy this page for additional entries, or use it as a guide for how to set up or adapt your own log.

WEEK 3 *FOOD LOG*

DATE	TIME	MEAL OR SNACK?	FOOD/DRINK	HUNGER (H) OR APPETITE (A)?	HUNGER 1–5	FULLNESS 1–5

Secrets of
Their
Success

**JAMES GRENO,
48**

WEIGHT LOST:
15 pounds*

James had been riding for 2 years when he started the BYBO plan. He was comfortable enough with his general riding ability to participate in local group rides in Pittsburgh. From a fitness standpoint, however, he felt stuck at the back of the pack. That all changed once he learned just how hard he could push himself—and how far it would get him.

One of his first messages to me, in fact, ended with "Those 3 minutes in Zone 4 is no fun!" That message, however, was followed by this one: "The high-intensity intervals are definitely improving my strength. I did a ride outside on Monday and when I got on the bike, my legs felt so strong, it felt like I had double my normal leg strength." Though that superhuman feeling dissipated after about 10 miles, he did get measurably faster in just a few weeks, improving his average speed by more than 1½ miles per hour on his usual route.

He also made the move from the back of the pack to the very front on his usual ride. "When we first started, I was always in the last half of the pack of some 35 to 40-some riders. On several of the last rides of the year I had moved up to third or fourth in the grouping and probably had a little more in the tank. When I realized where I was, I can't tell you how pumped I was."

Much of his improvement was physical, of course. But he also got mentally stronger. "I've grown in my ability to become comfortable with discomfort, and that to me is a big benefit physiologically. I'm doing hills that I would never have thought of doing before we began the program. At first I would say I was surviving the hills, whereas now I have a certain skill level that allows me to ride them with both confidence and a style where I am attacking the hill as opposed to surviving the punishment."

His cardiovascular fitness improved dramatically as well. "My heart rate went from what was a

Interestingly, James felt too light with that amount of weight loss and actually started eating more (healthy foods, that is) to put some weight back on. What a problem to have!

routine 185 beats per minute to never getting above 175, seemingly regardless of how much stress I put on myself."

On the food side, Jim got smarter. His diet wasn't bad, but he was cutting too far back on the carbs, which left him underfueled for his rides. He also simply wasn't eating enough and sometimes not often enough, grabbing a quick yogurt at 7:00 a.m. and not eating again until dinner at 6:00 p.m. Leslie implored him to pump up his morning meal by adding 1/4 cup of nuts, 1/3 cup of a Bear Naked granola, or some high-fiber cereal such as Fiber One to his morning yogurt. She also directed him to make at least one-fourth of his dinner carbohydrates by including foods like sweet potatoes, brown rice, or a little pasta so he had enough of the right energy sources for his rides.

"As the workouts intensify, you don't want to run out of steam, so just add a little tweak upward at meals and also include some snacks such as some nuts and dried fruit or a Lärabar or KIND bar, or a banana with 2 tablespoons of nut butter, if it's going to be many hours before your next meal," Leslie told him. Under her direction, Jim also started drinking more fluids and having a small carbohydrate/protein snack after hard rides.

He felt the effects instantly. "I was surprised that I was really able to feel the difference. Following an eating program allowed me to feel stronger and recover quicker. I'm now confident that I know how to fuel myself as I gear up for the upcoming season, when I'm planning on doing several different races already. I'm jazzed about that, as I've never done races before.

"On a larger level, I've developed an even greater appreciation for cycling and can't wait until we're able to get back outside in the early spring. Thank you for the time and energy you poured into the 12-week program. I owe you a beer (or wine). I'm looking forward to the rest of the journey."

CHAPTER 4

RULES
OF THE
ROAD

CARS. THAT'S THE BIGGEST fear of many new cyclists.
It's understandable. Motor vehicles weigh more
(a whole lot more) and travel faster (again, a whole lot
faster) than the bicycles with which they share the
roads. But, with knowledge and skill you *can* safely
and with confidence pilot your bike along most roads.
This week we'll focus on riding safely on all kinds
of roads and rides, improving the predictability of
your riding (which helps you be safe), and improving
your eating habits.

LIFE IN THE BIKE LANE (WHETHER OR NOT THERE'S A LANE)

I prefer to ride quiet, less-traveled roads where the occasional car having to
pass is no big deal. I certainly recommend you do the same. Of course, you
have to get to those quiet country roads, and for many of us (myself included)
that means negotiating through some town traffic.

Some towns, cities, and states have bike lanes. Most do not. Either way,
you have a right to ride on the road just like any other vehicle, with the exception of some high-speed highways, like major interstates you wouldn't want
to ride on anyway. The most important thing to remember is that when you
ride on the road, you follow the same rules as when you drive on the road.

First and foremost, ride on the right-hand side (or with the flow of traffic;
if you're in Australia or South Africa, for instance, you'll be on the left). Too
often new riders make the mistake of riding against traffic, thinking they're
safe because they can see oncoming cars. Nothing could be further from the
truth. Riding on the wrong side of the road is extremely unsafe and a leading
cause of bike-related accidents. Why? Physics. Let's say you're riding along
at 15 miles per hour, and oncoming traffic is flowing at 45 miles per hour. The

combined speed of you and any given car approaching you is 60 miles per hour. That leaves very little reaction time for either of you should something go awry (such as if you swerve to avoid a pothole). Now turn yourself around and ride the right way with the flow of traffic. Cars are now approaching you at just 30 miles per hour. Drivers have more time to see you and maneuver around you. You are also a more predictable part of the traffic flow. Statistically speaking, getting struck from behind while riding with the flow of traffic makes up a very small percentage of bike accidents. When you ride predictably, drivers can accommodate you.

So you know to ride on the right. But how far to the right? That depends. Obviously, if there's a bike lane, that's the place. If there isn't, you should ride as much on the shoulder as possible to allow cars to pass freely with a good bit of buffer room. If there is not much shoulder, you should ride a bit more into the lane rather than trying to squeeze onto two inches of pavement. Think of it this way: If you cram yourself onto the edge of the road, one, cars will be squeaking by you too close for comfort, and, two, you leave yourself no room to bail out should you need to move suddenly to miss an obstacle. By riding a bit more into the lane, you have a little bail-out room on the right and you're making drivers perform a clean pass around you, which results in more space between them and you as they come around.

If you're riding through a busy part of town where there are many parked cars on your right and traffic flowing on your left, do your best to create a healthy buffer between the two. As in the case where you have little shoulder, this means "taking the lane," or moving a bit into the flow of traffic. Riding too close to parked cars is dicey because it increases the likelihood of getting "doored," i.e., someone opening a car door right in your path. Give yourself some space and make a habit of looking into side-view mirrors and through rear windows to see if anyone might step out at any time. Also, don't weave in and out of the parking lane. Be predictable and ride a straight line down the lane where motorists can see and respond to you. It's far safer.

Just as you would signal your actions in a car, signal them on your bike so motorists know what you're doing. Keep your signals clear and simple. If you're turning right, stick your right arm out and point that way. If you're turning left, stick the left arm out. Yes, I know that technically you signal a right-hand turn with a bent left arm, but your average Joe and Jane behind the wheel don't know that and it's confusing. You want to be clear. Pointing in the direction you're going is clear. When you're coming to a stop, extend your left arm down at a diagonal with your palm facing back.

Negotiating intersections is probably the trickiest part of riding in traffic, especially when you need to cross through moving traffic to get into a turn lane (which shouldn't happen too often, but it does happen). Maneuver just as you would in a car. Look behind to find a break in the traffic and signal your move. Then move confidently over. I also like to make eye contact with motorists whenever possible to be sure that they see me. This is also true when I'm making a turn at an intersection. Eye contact is extremely helpful.

Along the lines of making eye contact and being seen, the more visible you are, the safer you are. Cycling clothes are often brightly colored and outfitted with reflective detailing for that reason. If you are going to be riding in low-light conditions (California's foggy mornings come to mind), definitely invest in some blinkies—small, flashing LED lights that you affix to your handlebars and seat tube (or any other nonmoving part on the back of your bike) that improve your visibility. Any bike shop will have them; they don't cost much and are a smart investment if you ride a lot.

Finally, be courteous. You are legally allowed to ride two abreast in many states, but that doesn't mean you always should. Common sense rules here. If you're on a busy road, ride single file so cars can pass more easily. Give cars room as you can. Don't cruise past a line of cars at a stop light, forcing cars to pass you again if they had trouble passing you the first time. You may occasionally encounter a mad motorist. Resist the urge to engage in a war of finger flipping and name-calling. It's not a battle you'll win, and it doesn't help the next cyclist who comes along. By and large, people are polite if you're polite to them.

ROAD HAZARDS

Certain road surfaces are inherently more dangerous to ride on. Here are some conditions to look for and suggestions on how to handle them.

PAINTED LINES. Road paint is important for marking lanes and other traffic control signals. Painted pavement is slippery when wet, so be especially careful if you have to cross it on rainy days. (For more on riding in the rain, see page 126.)

GRATES AND METAL COVERS. Storm sewer grates and manhole covers are often sunk into the road and can catch your wheels if you hit them improperly. They're also slippery when wet and best avoided entirely. Metal grate bridges are extremely slippery when wet, and I have seen a couple of nasty accidents on them when friends of mine skidded out in the rain. If you have to cross a metal grate bridge, ride straight and steady, and do not brake. If you don't feel confident, walk. It's better to be safe than scratched up.

RAILROAD TRACKS. Wet or dry (though especially when wet because they're slick), these can be a menace because they often run at odd angles and have many tire-grabbing grooves. To safely cross tracks, cross them as perpendicularly as possible and avoid slowing to a crawl. Your bike will clear bumps and obstacles more easily if you have a little momentum.

KICK UP YOUR CADENCE

When you watch the legs of a group of experienced cyclists spinning down the road, the first thing you'll notice (aside from all the sculpted calves and quads) is the briskness of their pedal stroke. Most seasoned cyclists aim for a cadence of about 90 revolutions per minute (rpm), meaning each foot completes one full circle 90 times in a minute.

A brisk cadence helps you ride safely and predictably, since it helps you maintain smooth forward momentum. It also keeps leg muscles fresh while keeping your cardiovascular system working at a fat-burning clip, so you can ride even longer before bonking (running out of energy). That being said, a high cadence doesn't come naturally to every cyclist. New riders especially tend to turn the pedals at a slower rate, partly because they haven't conditioned their neuromuscular and cardiovascular systems to pedal briskly and partly because they haven't mastered the art of pedaling. This week we'll work on both.

SPINNING CIRCLES

Picture-perfect pedaling is more than pushing down on the pedals. It's also pulling them up and around in an act that cyclists call pedaling circles. Ultimately, the goal is to eliminate any "dead spots" in your pedal stroke. At no point in each pedal stroke should your legs just be coming along for the ride; they should always be applying some pressure to propel you forward. The

TAKE A DRINK

Long rides mean drinking, maybe even eating, on the bike. I know riders who are so uncomfortable with the idea of reaching down for their water bottle and taking a drink that they simply won't do it. They'll get ragingly dehydrated and/or pull off and come to a complete stop somewhere to drink first. Both of those options toss a wet blanket on an otherwise good ride and are totally unnecessary because pulling out your water bottle, getting a drink, and putting the bottle back is a skill you can easily master with some practice.

In a parking lot or on a flat, grassy field, practice basic long-ride skills. Pull your water bottle from the cage, take a drink, and put it back without looking (or maybe just glancing down ever so briefly). Keep practicing until you can do it by feel. When you've got that dialed, practice reaching into the back pocket of your jersey and pulling out a snack. Both skills will go a long way toward increasing your riding pleasure.

smoother and more evenly powered your pedal stroke, the more efficient it is, which allows you to ride faster with less exertion.

Spinning circles is admittedly easier if you use clipless pedals (see page 72), which physically attach your foot to the pedal (it's not as scary as it sounds). Some riders instead use cages with toe straps, which bind your foot to the pedal, for the same effect. But even if you're riding in tennis shoes on plain flat pedals, you can still work on using your ankles to pull the pedal all away around the pedal stroke and minimize dead spots.

Here's a great description I got from Todd Carver, a biomechanics expert at Retül in Boulder, Colorado, who found that when riders pedaled using the following technique, they were able to produce the same amount of power (as measured in watts) at a heart rate that was about 5 beats per minute lower. Simply put: They rode the same speed with less work. This is how to do it.

ALIGN YOUR LEGS. Cyclists often refer to their legs as "pistons," and with good reason. From head-on, your legs should look like pistons firing straight up and down. Your knees should not flap from side to side. Your hips should not rock or wobble. If you have a chance, watch yourself pedal on a Spin bike or on your trainer in front of a mirror (or look down while pedaling in an open, untrafficked area). Your hips, knees, and ankles should line up throughout the pedal stroke. However, if you have bowed legs or other unique biomechanical characteristics, you may be an exception.

DROP YOUR HEEL OVER THE TOP. You produce the most power at the top of the pedal stroke, when your foot is in the 12 o'clock position. Maximize your power in that position by dropping your heel slightly as you come over the top of the stroke. Aim to have the heel of your foot parallel or just a bit below parallel as you start the downstroke.

SCRAPE THE SHOE. As you come through the bottom of the stroke, engage your calf muscles and pull through, pointing your toes down slightly. Seasoned cyclists often recommend visualizing scraping mud off the bottom of your shoe.

BRING YOUR KNEES TO THE BARS. Everyone loses a little momentum and power on the upstroke. This is also where some people's knees swing out to the side. Minimize that by consciously working on an active upstroke. As you begin to come across the top of the stroke, visualize driving your knee forward toward the bar. Be sure to keep your pelvis rock steady in the saddle throughout the whole stroke so there's no wasted energy.

A QUICK (AND FAT-BURNING) CADENCE

Now that you've gotten the hang of (or are at least practicing) spinning circles, let's work on spinning them briskly. First, determine your current revolutions per minute. To do so, simply count how many times your right foot swings down toward the ground over 30 seconds and multiply by 2.

Your optimal pedal cadence depends upon myriad factors, including your muscle fiber composition, the type of cycling you're doing, your gear, and even your age. When you spin at a very high cadence (say, 100 rpm or above) in a moderately light gear, you rely mostly on your aerobic, fat-burning energy system to do the work. Low cadences (say, below 80 rpm) in bigger gears use more muscle fibers and tap into the anaerobic system that burns glycogen (stored carbs). That's why most of us find the pedaling sweet spot—where we're neither frying our muscles nor wearing ourselves out—between those two ends of the spectrum. Most coaches recommend about 90 rpm. It's not a magic number by any means, but it's worth practicing picking up your pedaling speed if your cadence is below 80 rpm.

WORKOUTS FOR // WEEK 4

WORKOUT: CRANK THE CADENCE

// **SKILL DRILL:** Spin-Ups

Spin at your normal cadence (whatever comes naturally without thinking about it) for 45 seconds. Then, staying seated, speed up as much as you can without bouncing around on the saddle for 15 seconds. Repeat 3 to 5 times. Ideally you should do this in a parking lot or on an empty stretch of road so you don't have to worry about traffic.

THE BYBO RIDE

TERRAIN: Flat to undulating

WHAT TO DO	INTENSITY	HOW LONG
Warmup	ZONE 1–2	~15 min
Speed up to 90–100 rpm*	ZONE 2–3	~1 min
Pedal at your normal speed	ZONE 2	~2 min
Pedal fast (> 100 rpm if possible)**	ZONE 3	~1 min
Pedal ~your normal speed	ZONE 2	~2 min
Repeat the sequence (minus the warmup) 2 more times		
Pedal slightly faster than your normal speed	ZONE 2	~10 min

Finish with easy pedaling going home.

TOTAL TIME: ~45 min

Perform this workout 3 times this week.

NOTE: *If you're already riding for longer than 45 minutes, simply extend the beginning or end of your ride or add another interval sequence.*

TAKE HOME: If you've been riding at a very slow (e.g., 60 rpm) cadence, higher speeds will feel extremely unnatural at first, and you may not be able to hit 90 or 100 rpm during the drills. Keep at it. Before long you'll notice that a brisker cadence (e.g., over 80 rpm) feels like less work in the long run, so riding is more enjoyable and longer rides more achievable. This workout will help make those higher cadences feel more comfortable, as well as teach you how to manipulate your cadence to control your effort.

*You may need to shift into an easier gear to do this. Your heart rate will go up, but your legs should not be burning.

**Don't sacrifice proper form during this segment of the workout. If you start rocking at the hips or flailing at the knees, slow down until you're in control.

THE INSIDE RIDE

Similar to last week, this workout incorporates cardioresistance training, which blends cardio and strength training into the same workout. Once again, we'll mimic the outdoor ride and concentrate on achieving a quick cadence. If you're doing this workout on a traditional Spin bike (i.e., one in a gym with a weighted flywheel), it's *very* easy to do high-cadence drills because the weight of the flywheel helps you pick up speed and maintain momentum. You should still feel the change in your cardiovascular effort as you ramp up your pedaling speed. And the same form rules apply as for outdoor riders: If your form starts falling apart, with your knees flailing and/or your hips rocking, bring down the pace until you're back in control.

WHAT TO DO	INTENSITY	HOW LONG
Warmup	ZONE 1–2	~10 min
Speed up to 90–100 rpm*	ZONE 2–3	~1 min
Pedal ~your normal speed	ZONE 2	~2 min
Pedal fast (> 100 rpm if possible)**	ZONE 3	~1 min
Pedal ~your normal speed	ZONE 2	~2 min
Repeat the sequence (minus the warmup)		
Pedal ~your normal speed, easing off for the final 30 sec	ZONE 2 to 1	~1 min

Dismount and perform the BYBO Core Workout, then repeat the circuit.

Get back on the bike, spin for ~2 min, and repeat the entire fast pedaling and Core Workout sequence once more (but do the Core Workout just once through this time).

Finish with some easy stretching after you're done with the core moves.

TOTAL TIME: ~40 min

You may need to reduce your resistance to do this. Your heart rate will go up, but your legs should not be burning.

**Don't sacrifice proper form during this segment. If you start rocking at the hips or flailing at the knees, slow down until you're in control.*

WORKOUT LOG

Please log your workouts for the week.

WEEK 4				
BYBO Rides (including pleasure cruise) and Core Workouts	Date: Notes:	Date: Notes:	Date: Notes:	Date: Notes:
Cross-training and/or rest	Date: Activity: Duration:	Date: Activity: Duration:	Date: Activity: Duration:	Date: Activity: Duration:

ANY OBSTACLES? _____

ACCOMPLISHMENTS? _____

OTHER NOTES: _____

BYBO CORE WORKOUT

(SEE PAGE 24 FOR EXERCISE DIRECTIONS)

Do the moves one after another like a circuit. Then repeat.

* Plank
* Spider

* Bridge
* Dip

BYBO STRETCHES

(SEE PAGE 36 FOR EXERCISE STRETCH DIRECTIONS)

* Figure 4
* Stork
* Windshield Wiper

* Cobra
* Prayer Pose

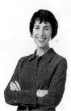

LESLIE'S LESSONS

BIKE YOUR BUTT OFF! EATING PLAN: HABITS, ACCOUNTABILITY, AND PORTIONS

By now you're a few weeks into this plan. You've been logging your food, gauging your hunger, spacing your meals properly, and stocking your fridge. All of that is great! But I'm betting there is still room for improvement.

Do you do any of the following?

* Eat more on the weekend than during the week?
* Eat a different number of meals on weekends or off days than during the week?
* Consume a lot of calories in beverages?

* Eat really fast?
* Eat or drink standing up?
* Eat in the car?
* Eat while watching TV or at the computer?

If the answer is yes to any of these, what can and will you change?

The body really wants consistency if you are going to be successful with weight loss and management. So pick a number of meals and a calorie level and try to make it a 7-day effort. Also try to space your intake more evenly over the day rather than eating a little at one time and a lot at others.

Could your beverages be lighter (in calories, that is)? If you don't chew, you won't be as satisfied, and honestly, what is there to chew in sweetened tea or cider or beer? That doesn't mean drinking only water, but it does mean making some compromise, such as having three parts water to one part juice or a smaller glass of undiluted juice. Pick the option that is most satisfying to you.

What's the rate of your eating? There's a reason I have asked you to log the time it takes you to eat. We are not awarding prizes for being the first one done. You want to be successful with weight management? S-L-O-W D-O-W-N. Put the brake on the plate. Put the utensil or food down between bites. Chew. Swallow. Pick up the utensil or food and repeat. If you do this, it will take you longer to eat, you will feel fuller, you will be less likely to overconsume. For those of you who are already slow eaters, keep it up, but for the hares among you, I want you to grow a shell and become a tortoise at the table!

What about how you eat? If you are one of those people who stands at the fridge, in front of the cabinet, or over the kitchen sink, *stop it*! Sit in a chair at a table, eating off the bowl or plate, so you know what you are doing. Again, pay more attention to what you do; it will translate to a slimmer you!

As mentioned, location is key. Do not eat in the car while your eyes and mind are necessarily distracted. This is all about self-accountability and changing habits. I prefer that you pay full attention to your food. If you must multitask while you eat, how about listening to calming music while catching up on some reading? It will slow you down and be a more enjoyable experience.

BE ACCOUNTABLE!

At the end of the day, the only one who knows what, when, and how much you put in your mouth is you. That is the way it should be, and although having your support system and an eating confidant is not a bad idea, you need to do what is best for you. Some people are stealth dieters and don't want anyone else to know; others do better when they involve a family member or friend. Logging your intake is a great way to create accountability. So is planning your eating and creating a shopping list and sticking to both.

PORTION CONTROL

This is the main focus of the week. If you don't currently own measuring cups and spoons, go to a dollar store and pick some up. Why? Humor me and try this little experiment at home. Get out your favorite breakfast cereal, or the rice or pasta you would have at dinner, and pour or plate your regular portion. Then look at the box or container and see what the serving size actually is and how close you are with your typical amount. Who knew that a serving of Grape-Nuts is ½ cup? That barely covers the bottom of the cereal bowl. If you have a scale, use it! If not, use the information on the Nutrition Facts panel to determine the serving size; when you buy meat, chicken, or fish, you can ask the butcher to portion it for you.

What about eating out? Well, many restaurants are trying to serve the right sizes, but you still have to pay attention. Here are my recommendations.

- Ask for an appetizer portion of an entrée.

- Ask if the restaurant offers half portions.

- Share meals.

- Ask for half the entrée to be brought to the table, and the rest packed up for another meal.

- In general, eat only a hand-size amount (a woman's hand, a man's palm) of chicken, fish, or meat.

- You want two fists' worth of vegetables.

- One tightly balled fist is the right amount of rice, pasta, or potato.

- Back away from descriptions such as "bottomless," "free refills," and "monster."

And let's not forget about what is in the glass. If the server asks if you want a small or large drink, the correct answer is small. If the margarita is the size of your head, you better be sharing it with five other people. Alcoholic beverages, sweetened tea, and regular soda can often be deal breakers when you are trying to lose weight.

This week, the food log is simple. I want you to keep track of your eating speed (rate), what you eat and drink, and the portion sizes as best you can. Below, you'll find an example of what form your chart should follow.

WEEK 4 *FOOD LOG*

DATE	RATE	FOOD	DRINK	AMOUNT

CHAPTER 5

KEEP
ON
ROLLING

THIS WASN'T THE FIRST time Jaime Livingood had taken up cycling. In fact, there had been several tries. But each time, it fizzled out soon after it started. She just never felt completely comfortable on her bike; she fell more than she cared to admit and didn't know how to ride in a way that made her crave cycling. So time after time, she'd start with a bang only to end up slowly but surely racking her bike in a corner somewhere, and its tires deflating just as her motivation had.

This time was different. For one, she started from scratch, homing in on mastering the very basics—starting, stopping, turning, getting a drink without wobbling, and so forth. She gained confidence. This led her to take advantage of one of cycling's most wonderful benefits—she found friends to ride with. In her own words:

> I just wanted to drop you a little note about how great my first group ride was last night. Liz, our ride leader, went over a few basics and then took me and two other girls on a night ride.
>
> I was nervous all day. It started to drizzle on the way to the shop, which made me more uneasy. After Liz talked to us about night riding, off we went. I had a combo of running and cycling clothes to keep me warm, which was key for sure. I think I need to start getting some more clothing going forward. I was nervous, but I felt like I heard you in the back of my head giving me direction on turning and pedaling and finding my happy gear place. I stopped focusing on the ground right in front of my front wheel and just enjoyed the company and talking with the two other new gals I met.
>
> I have no idea how fast we were going and it was flat. But I know

that we did just over 9 miles. I don't think I could have done that without your coaching, and I just needed to tell you that. I am falling in love with my bike all over again and all I want to do is get back on my bike again! I am not sure I have had this feeling since I was 12 and rode my bike everywhere.

Liz promises that she will take us out on more night rides (and more rides in general)—so I am going to hold her to it! But I just wanted to thank you for getting me on your plan.

This week we'll focus on all those key elements—from finding cycling buddies to increasing your confidence—that will keep you rolling (because you really want to!) long after the novelty of being on a new "exercise plan" has worn off.

BIRDS OF A FEATHER

Remember when you were a kid and wanted to go out and play? You'd call a bunch of friends, bang on doors, hunt around the cul-de-sac looking for someone to shoot hoops, skateboard, bike, or generally run around with. If you found a friend or two, you'd be out for hours, maybe long past when you were supposed to be home. You probably even lost track of time. But if no one was around? You were more likely to toss a few baskets, then head back home and slump in front of the TV because, whether you're 11 or 41, playing with other people is far more fun.

Riding is similar. Sure, there are plenty of times when I love to take a spin by myself to think through some work problems—or clear my head of them. But even though I love, love, love riding my bike, there are plenty of times when my motivation to change clothes and head out the door is low if I'm going out alone. That's why one way to ensure a long, rich cycling life is to find some riding friends who'll join you to go out and play, at least from time to time.

What's more, it's actually easier to ride with other people not only because time flies while you're out there chatting, but also because when you're with a few other riders, you can share the work and get a break from the wind by taking turns riding behind one another in what's known as a paceline. Riding behind other riders is called drafting, and it can reduce how much you have to work at any given pace by up to 30 percent.

A great resource for finding riding friends is your local bike shop. Chances are it has regular shop rides for riders of similar fitness levels and goals. Group rides are generally categorized by pace and intensity, including A rides, which go really fast and will "drop" you (leave you behind) if you can't keep up; B rides, which are steady and brisk, keeping everyone together; and C rides, which are superrelaxed and casual. You can pick the one that best fits your wants and needs.

Most casual rides are very welcoming to newbies and the riders will happily give you some pointers on riding in a group. The most important thing is to know how to behave in a paceline (a single- or double-file line of riders). Here are some basic rules that will help you ride with others smoothly *and* safely.

BE PREDICTABLE. Hold your line. Avoid sudden braking, swerving, and accelerating. Stay loose and relaxed. If you see potholes or other obstacles in the road, call them out for the riders behind you. Likewise, indicate when you're turning, slowing, or stopping. Communication is key to keep the group going smoothly and safely.

GIVE SPACE. You want to follow the rider in front of you closely, but have enough room to react to changes in pace. For experienced cyclists, it's inches, not feet. If you're 3 feet behind someone, you're not really in a paceline. That's a gap. If you are are new to pacelines, try half a wheel to a wheel's worth of space.

LOOK AHEAD. Behave as you would when driving in traffic. You don't just stare at the car directly in front of you. You look down the road to see what traffic is doing ahead. The same rule applies when riding in a line. Don't fixate on the wheel in front of you. Look ahead, through the rider in front of you, so you can see the other riders and the road and anticipate what the group will do and react to the terrain.

KEEP THE PACE. Maintain the general pace of the group. Stay even with the rider next to you if in a double paceline. If you're too tired to work at the front, stay in the back of the pack. As you ride, adjust your speed to maintain a constant effort within the group. Try to avoid pedaling like mad and then coasting. It creates a yo-yo effect in the group. Instead, make minute adjustments in how hard you're pressing down on the pedals. Gently feather your brakes while you pedal. Stick your head out in the wind a bit. All these will temper your speed without your surging or stalling within the line.

When it's your turn at the front, keep the speed steady. Some riders unwittingly crank up the pace when they take the lead. Don't. Keep the pace the same as it's been (a speedometer is helpful here). Stay at the front only as long as you feel comfortable, but not more than a few minutes. Then pull off and decelerate without completely slowing down. Another common error is pulling off and slowing *way* down as the pack goes by. Then you have to push too hard to catch back up. Instead, pedal moderately fast, staying relatively close to the riders passing by (this helps you stay in their draft), and rejoin the pack after the last rider comes by.

MORE TOYS AND ACCESSORIES

We said it before, and we'll say it again. Cycling is a gear-happy sport. I'll be the first to say that the right equipment and accessories can definitely make you even happier on your bike, especially as you ride farther and longer in a wider variety of conditions. Here are a few items worth checking out to enhance your cycling experience.

GPS. Beware. Once you try a cycling GPS navigation unit, such as those by Garmin, you won't ever want to ride without one. These dashboards for your bike are easier to use than standard bike computers (there's no sensor or calibration necessary; just turn it on and go) and deliver far more information. At a glance you can see how many feet of elevation you've climbed, the temperature, number of calories burned, even where you are if you buy one with maps installed. Garmins also make it easy to track your progress over time. You can plug them into your home computer and download your rides using programs like Garmin Connect and Strava.

ARM WARMERS. These removable sleeves may be my favorite piece of cycling attire. Why? Because I don't have to debate whether to wear short sleeves and be chilly for a while or long sleeves and bake for a while when I'm doing a ride that starts at 9:00 a.m., when the temperature is about 60°F, and ends 2 hours later, when it can easily be 10° or 15°F warmer. I slip on my arm warmers to start the ride and peel them off and put them in my pocket when the day and my body heat up.

VEST. Because your torso is relatively inactive and you generate a lot of wind as you slice through the air, it's easy for your core to get cold even on a fairly warm spring or autumn day. Like arm warmers, a vest can make the difference between riding in comfort and sucking it up and being cold when the temperature hovers in that in-between zone where a jacket is more than you need. They also serve as nice protection against the wind on long downhill stretches.

KNEE WARMERS. Knee warmers and their full-length counterpart, leg warmers, turn any pair of cycling shorts into knickers (to keep your knees warm) or tights (to keep the entire length of your legs warm) and are considerably less expensive than knickers or tights. If you plan to ride when the temperature is lower than 65 degrees, a set of knee warmers is a smart investment. Cold knees are achy knees. (And nobody needs achy knees.)

SHOE COVERS. Cycling shoes (and the tennis or running shoes you might be wearing) are generally well ventilated to keep your feet cool while you're generating heat exercising. That's great until the weather gets cold. Shoe covers slip over your cycling shoes, keeping out the cold air and holding in the warmth of your feet. Fair-weather riders don't need shoe covers. Those who pedal year-round very much appreciate them.

SADDLEBAG. Sure you have jersey pockets to put all your stuff into. But let's face it, it gets old stuffing your shirt full of tubes, levers, and such. A saddlebag— a small pack that straps onto the rails beneath your seat—lets you carry it all on your bike, leaving your pockets free for other essentials. A well-stocked saddlebag also gives you one less thing to think about. You have all your repair items ready to go. You can just saddle up and ride.

MIRRORS. Mirrors are a controversial cycling accessory. Some riders swear by rearview mirrors that you can attach to your handlebars, helmet, and/or glasses. Others dislike mirrors because they feel they can distract cyclists from the road ahead, don't offer a wide enough field of vision, and can be dangerous if cyclists rely on them rather than physically looking back over their shoulders to be sure all is clear before turning or switching lanes. If a mirror makes you feel safer and that helps you ride more, by all means pick one up. Just remember, it doesn't replace scanning for traffic over your shoulder.

WORKOUT: TEMPO TIME!

Tempo, or "steady state," riding means riding at a pace that is right above your aerobic comfort zone, but not quite at your threshold (the point at which your muscles scream Uncle! if you stay there too long). I tell people to imagine they are riding with a slightly faster friend. They can still speak in short sentences. They're not gasping. But they're working fairly hard and going faster than they would on their own. That's tempo. Riding at tempo helps bump up your fitness, strength, and endurance. It also prepares you to join more spirited group rides, which often require a bit of tempo riding to hang with the pack.

// SKILL DRILL: Smooth and Steady

Tempo riding requires you to be smooth and steady. Practice keeping your upper body relaxed and quiet so you don't waste energy. Then focus on your pedal stroke and on spinning those perfect, smooth circles that we practiced last week while working on cadence. Concentrate on pulling up with your legs, bringing your knees up toward the handlebars on each revolution, so that you use all your muscles evenly to propel the bike forward. This exercise is easier with clipless pedals (or toe straps) because you are physically attached to the pedals, but you can do it with flat pedals as well.

THE BYBO RIDE

TERRAIN: Flat to gently undulating

WHAT TO DO	INTENSITY	HOW LONG
Warmup	ZONE 1–2	15 min
Increase pace/intensity	ZONE 2	10 min
Increase pace/intensity to tempo	ZONE 3	10 min
Ease back on the intensity	ZONE 1–2	2–5 min
Increase pace/intensity to tempo	ZONE 3	10 min

Ease back and finish with easy pedaling going home.

TOTAL TIME: 55–60 min

Perform this workout 3 times this week.

TAKE HOME: This workout conditions your lungs and legs to withstand the challenges of maintaining a steady effort and gets you ready to meet the demands of longer, harder rides.

NOTE: *If you're already riding for longer than 55 to 60 minutes, simply extend the beginning or end of your ride or add another tempo sequence.*

THE INSIDE RIDE

Similar to last week, this workout incorporates cardioresistance training, which blends cardio and strength training in the same workout. Once again, we'll mimic the outdoor ride and concentrate on getting in and out of the saddle to build fitness.

WHAT TO DO	INTENSITY	HOW LONG
Warmup	ZONE 1–2	2–3 min
Steady, brisk, moderate resistance	ZONE 2	10 min
Increase resistance to simulate a moderate hill; stay smooth	ZONE 2–3*	2 min
Pick up your pace	ZONE 3	2 min.
Increase resistance a bit and stand, picking up the pace as though cresting a climb	ZONE 3	30–60 sec
Sit back down, lower resistance, ease off the effort	ZONE 2 to 1	2 min

Dismount and perform the BYBO Core Workout.

Get back on the bike, spin for 2–3 min, and repeat the hill climb sequence once more (but do the Core Workout circuit just once this time).

Finish with some easy stretching after you're done with the core moves.

TOTAL TIME: ~50 min

This effort should feel like it's on the breaking point between aerobic and hard.

WORKOUT LOG

Please log your workouts for the week.

WEEK 5				
BYBO Rides (including pleasure cruise) and Core Workouts	Date: Notes:	Date: Notes:	Date: Notes:	Date: Notes:
Cross-training and/or rest	Date: Activity: Duration:	Date: Activity: Duration:	Date: Activity: Duration:	Date: Activity: Duration:

ANY OBSTACLES? _____

ACCOMPLISHMENTS? _____

OTHER NOTES: _____

BYBO CORE WORKOUT

(SEE PAGE 24 FOR EXERCISE DIRECTIONS)

Do the moves one after another like a circuit. Then repeat. Note: New moves this week!

* Crank Plank
* Spiderman Pushup

* Figure 4 Bridge
* Tipping Bird

BYBO STRETCHES

(SEE PAGE 36 FOR STRETCH DIRECTIONS)

* Figure 4
* Stork
* Windshield Wiper

* Cobra
* Prayer Pose

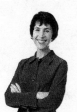

LESLIE'S LESSONS

BIKE YOUR BUTT OFF! EATING PLAN: STAYING ON TRACK AND FUELING FOR THE RIDE

I don't want you to derail, whether or not you are on the trail, so let's talk about those hidden saboteurs that are the roadblocks to healthful eating.

HEALTH HALO FOODS. Research shows that people tend to overeat foods that they perceive as virtuous, such as those that are organic, natural, have no added sugars, and are fat-free. Let's take a look at what those labels mean and why they don't give you a free pass to eat with abandon.

* The designation "organic," by law, specifies that no pesticides in produce or on grains, or foods that contain no antibiotics or hormones, or the animal's feed contains no hormones or antibiotics. That is all well and good, but organic gummy bears are not any better for you than nonorganic ones.

* The same goes for "natural." Natural peanut butter still has the same amounts of calories and fat as any other peanut butter.

* "No added sugars" does not mean *no sugar.* It means that the sugar in the product is there naturally, such as in fruit juice or applesauce. So don't think that you will always realize a significant calorie savings.

* "Fat-free" *does not* mean calorie-free, and often these foods are higher in sugar and/or salt because if you take out the fat, you have to put something else in there to provide taste.

THINKING THAT IF YOU EAT A SMALL AMOUNT IT WON'T COUNT. News flash—Hershey's Kisses are adorable, but if you wolf down half a bag, the calories add up, my friend. If you're going to eat a small amount, truly eat a small amount, by putting a small serving on a dish, putting the bag or box away, and enjoying your treat.

FORGETTING ABOUT THE LIQUID CALORIES. The more you ride, the thirstier you might be, but think before you drink. It is way too easy to chug several hundred calories in sports beverages, beer, fruit punch, sweetened tea, and/or soda. So be careful and consider the calories in the glass when you figure out your calories for the day. Just because you don't chew drinks doesn't mean they are freebies!

And while we are talking about fluids, a word about alcohol. Alcohol is an appetite stimulant, which means if you drink, you may be hungrier, and usually not for a bag of carrots! The closest you may get to a vegetable is the Bloody Mary mix and celery stalk. Alcohol itself has calories, what you mix it with may have calories (even tonic water—the same number of calories as a cola beverage), and the alcohol may make you consume more calories, so be aware.

KEEPING TEMPTING FOODS AROUND. Everybody has a food or several that they have a hard time controlling their intake of. Really now, are you going to eat only a couple of chips, or one small scoop of ice cream? Don't rely on willpower. Get the temptation out of your house, desk drawer, gym bag, or wherever it calls your name from.

ON THE BIKE

So let's switch gears and talk about fueling and hydration for your rides. The goal is to prepare, prefuel, and prehydrate so you can go faster, longer, and stronger. That being said, amounts and timing, as well as choices, are critical. (And please note, we are talking about longer and harder rides here. If you're going out for an easy 30 minutes to an hour, you can just saddle up and roll!) In general, strive for 16 to 20 ounces of liquid 1 hour before you ride.

All beverages except alcohol will work to hydrate you, but carbonated beverages stay in your stomach longer, so the fluid is not as readily available. Concentrated beverages such as sweetened energy drinks and fruit drinks also take longer to leave your stomach and contain a lot of calories. The best bets are water, a diluted sports drink, or a lower-sugar sports drink. It takes about 60 minutes for 20 ounces of fluid to leave your stomach, so time your drinking according to when you ride. Even if you are a heavy sweater, there is no need to drink a gallon before you mount your bike. But a sip won't work either, so get in the habit of training your guts, and consider the drinking to be a part of your warmup.If you don't drink, it gets harder to drink enough when you're riding because your body is now playing catchup.

What about preride fuel? I am not a big fan of riding on empty because this forces your body to use its own muscle as a fuel source. Unacceptable. But don't overdo it. The key is *less* is *more*. You don't need a lot of fuel before your ride. You need just enough to top off your energy stores.

A small amount, such as a quarter of a peanut butter sandwich, a small banana with 1 tablespoon nut butter, $\frac{1}{4}$ cup trail mix, a cup of cereal and milk, or a Greek yogurt with 2 tablespoons of granola will all do the trick.

And when should you eat? About 30 to 60 minutes before getting on the bike. Again, this is only if you'll be riding for more than an hour, you will be riding hard, or you haven't eaten anything in a few hours. No need to nosh before an easy pleasure ride.

WHAT ABOUT DURING RIDES?

For 1 hour of cycling, water alone is fine, but once you get into longer times and distances, you need to be consuming some fuel on the bike. That is when a sports drink or products such as gels, chews, honey sticks, or sugar cubes come in handy. On average, most people need only about 30 grams of carbohydrates per hour of riding after the first hour. So pick *one* of the following per hour:

* 16 ounces sports drink
* 1 gel pack
* 4 chews

* 1 tablespoon honey or 3 honey sticks
* 6 to 8 sugar cubes

WHAT ABOUT HYDRATION?

You need to drink according to your sweat rate, especially when it's hot outside. Drinking a bottle an hour generally is a good ballpark amount, but it's helpful to know your personal sweat rate so you can stay hydrated on long, hot rides.

The easiest way is to use the following sweat rate calculator. All you need to do is weigh yourself before and after you ride.

SWEAT RATE CALCULATOR

Preride weight – postride weight in ounces (there are 16 ounces in a pound)

+

The number of ounces of fluid you drank during your ride (look on the bottle)

÷

The number of hours you rode

=

Your hourly sweat rate or the number of ounces of fluid you need to drink per hour

EXAMPLE

180 pounds – 178 pounds = 2 pounds, or 32 ounces

+

20 ounces

÷

2-hour ride

32 ounces + 20 ounces = 52 ounces ÷ 2 hours =
26 ounces of fluid required per hour

Again, you need to practice taking in the fluid while you ride, which means it must be available, and also try to consume gulps instead of sips when riding. Larger volumes of fluid leave the stomach faster, so you won't feel bloated.

After your ride, you need to drink 24 ounces of fluid for every pound you have lost, but you can consume this extra liquid over the rest of the day.

So if you are being mindful of calories, opt for water or a lower-sugar sports drink during the ride and remember, after the second hour, it is either the sports drink or the gels/chews/honey sticks/sugar cubes and water, but not both a sports drink and another carbohydrate supplement.

FOR THE SALTY SWEATERS AMONG US

Does your sweat sting your eyes, taste salty in your mouth, or make your skin feel gritty? Are there white streaks on your jersey and shorts or on the inside of your cap? That is salt.

Those who are salty sweaters are more prone to muscle cramping, so you should not drink water exclusively. Sports drinks do contain sodium to help offset the losses, and since most of you are not going to chug salty V8 juice when you ride, you can add $\frac{1}{2}$ teaspoon of salt to 32 ounces of sports drink—just shake it up before you drink it to disperse the salt.

WHAT ABOUT SOME EXTRA ENERGY?

Red Bull, 5-Hour Energy Shots, and espresso are common sights in cycling circles. Caffeine is a stimulant, not a source of fuel for energy. That doesn't mean you shouldn't use it, but 5-Hour Energy Shots contain 5 calories and only 1 ounce of liquid and 150 milligrams of caffeine. That is one rotation of the wheels and you're done. You need more of both fuel and fluid.

If you want to use caffeine, it is important to understand that it is a central nervous system stimulant. That's a good thing, since it can make you feel like you're "raring to go." And caffeine has been shown to be a performance-enhancing substance. Just use it with care. Because it is a stimulant, it can cause your heart to race and your breathing to speed up, especially if you're sensitive to it. It may also have a laxative effect.

So limit yourself to a cup or two an hour or so before you ride. Also, we're talking black coffee (or coffee with a splash of milk) here, not high-calorie coffee drinks with added syrups, sugars, whipped cream, and/or cream that can add tons of calories and take hours of riding to burn off. Also, read your labels. A regular Red Bull has 80 milligrams of caffeine but packs 120 calories.

YOUR TRACKING ASSIGNMENT THIS WEEK

This week, keep track of what you do in terms of fueling and hydrating before, during, and after rides, and also determine your sweat rate so you can drink the appropriate amount.

HOURLY SWEAT RATE AND AMOUNT OF FLUID TO CONSUME HOURLY DURING RIDES

Preride weight – postride weight in ounces

+

Fluid consumed during rides in ounces

÷

Number of hours you ride

=

Hourly sweat rate

My preride food preferences:

My preferences during rides:

Secrets of Their Success

CAROL MALAZITA, 56

WEIGHT LOST:
15 pounds, plus 4 inches off her waist

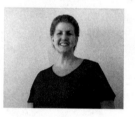

Carol came to us tired of the weight-loss roller coaster that she'd been riding for the past 20 years. Her biggest problem: She hated to exercise. Making matters worse, she'd also had some health issues, including several abdominal surgeries and stress fractures in her feet from dance classes and treadmill workouts, that made many traditional exercise plans painful.

"I have done Jenny Craig, Nutrisystem, and Weight Watchers over the past 20 years. I was successful to a point in that I could lose the 20 to 30 pounds that I needed to lose, but I then would put back on the weight little by little because I never really established an exercise program that I could stick with and I eat very poorly," she recalls. "I decided I could tackle bike riding, even with stress fractures in my feet. As long as I wear the orthotics in my sneakers, I'm good to go."

And go she did. Her first step was joining the Y, going there directly after leaving the middle school where she teaches French and German. "I used to come home and start eating from the time I walked in the door and began cooking dinner to bedtime. It occurred to me that I didn't need to do that," she says. "So I stop at the gym first. I see my students, and we're all there huffing and puffing and being healthy. It's a good thing."

Carol thrived on the structure and specificity of the program. "I liked that it gave me instruction on how hard I should be working and for how long," she explains. For her, the four core moves were life altering. "My abdominals had gotten very weak from all the surgeries. I couldn't even get out of bed without rolling over and pushing myself up with my arms. I kept thinking I was too young to feel this old. Thanks to the exercises, I can get out of bed normally again. That's a big deal."

On the food side, Carol didn't completely overhaul her eating, but rather cleaned it up and learned to practice portion control. "Restaurants were always a challenge, but I shared dessert and counted out six french fries rather than eating the whole pile on my plate," she says. Following Leslie's suggestion, she also tried to add protein to all her meals.

"I noticed Carol would eat more carb-focused foods such as parfait, apples, pretzels, blueberry biscuits, and Cheerios some days, and other days would eat more protein-focused foods like Greek yogurt, turkey, and shrimp salad. I said, let's combine those to get the best of both worlds every day," recalls Leslie, who instructed Carol to get protein in the form of yogurt, eggs, cottage cheese, fish, poultry, or meat at every meal along with some carb, like a quarter of a small potato, half a cup of rice, half a cup of pasta, or a slice of bread.

The close attention to eating balanced, well-portioned meals worked. The pounds came off steadily—even over the Thanksgiving holidays. "I can't believe I lost weight over the holidays. But it was great. I wasn't stuffed. I wasn't uncomfortable. I wasn't unhappy with myself. I had a great meal, and I stopped eating when I'd had enough. What a concept!"

The one-two punch of getting stronger and shedding pounds has left Carol feeling better than she has in years. "My back doesn't hurt. My knees don't hurt. I feel great and have lots of energy. The biggest change is how much I enjoy it all. I used to hate exercise. Now I really like it," she says. "It's changed my life."

CHAPTER 6

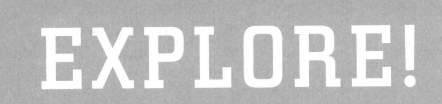

EXPLORE!

HANDS DOWN, ONE OF the biggest joys of riding a bike is the ability to go places you wouldn't ordinarily go and see even familiar neighborhoods in a whole different light. You can cover more ground riding your bike than you can walking, and you can coast and look around more than you can behind a steering wheel. So this week, I invite you to take some new roads and paths.

Is there a park you drive by regularly but have never ridden in? Take your bike and spin around it. How about all those side streets in your neighborhood? You might be surprised by the quirky, fun lawn ornaments and outdoor decorations you may discover. Ride down a road you generally pass by just because. Some of my favorite routes have come about because I or one of my riding friends said, "Huh, I wonder where that goes?"

HIT THE DIRT

If you have a mountain bike, take it on some new trails. Riding rougher terrain can be exhilarating and make you feel like a kid again. I'm not talking about hucking your bike off of 3-foot ledges, jumping massive logs, or riding treacherous rock gardens—there are books devoted to that if you want to give it a whirl. But any mountain bike can handle some small rocks and roots. And it's fun. Here are some fundamentals that will keep you rolling.

RIDE WITHIN YOURSELF. The first rule of trail riding is to ride within yourself, i.e., don't get in over your head. Think of it like skiing: You'd never in a million runs take the lift to the top and drop onto a double black diamond slope your first time down the mountain. The same is true for off-road riding. Mountain bike trails range in difficulty from wide, flat cinder paths to rutted, rocky, near-vertical descents. Your best bet is to get the feeling for off-road riding on a nearby bridle trail or smooth dirt path. As you become more comfortable, venture onto some rougher terrain, like rocky or wooded *singletrack* (a hiking-type trail usually strewn with rocks, roots, and water crossings). Remember, anytime you feel outside your comfort zone, you can get off the bike and walk.

LOOK WHERE YOU WANT TO GO. If you remember nothing else, remember this one. Your bike will follow your eyes. Point them where you want to go. There are plenty of things on the trail you don't want to hit—rocks, ditches, roots—don't fixate on them! Fix your gaze on the smoothest line ahead of your tires. Mountain bikers refer to this coveted path of least resistance as "the line." The more you ride, the better you'll be able to pick your lines and ride smoothly around and through obstacles of all kinds.

BALANCE YOUR WEIGHT. Your front tire needs just enough weight to stay grounded, but not so much that it can't freely move over obstacles in the way. Mountain bikes are designed for fat tires and have shock absorbers that allow you to roll over small to midsize obstacles on the trail. Avoid leaning too heavily on your handlebars. Instead, keep your weight evenly distributed between your hands, feet, and butt. As you approach an obstacle on the trail, lift up on the bars to pull the front tire up and over whatever is in the way. After your front tire clears the obstacle, lift your butt off the saddle to unweight your back tire so it can clear it as well. When you're going down steep descents, place your butt way back to allow your front wheel to roll freely while keeping the rear wheel planted firmly on the ground.

MAINTAIN MOMENTUM. Mountain biking follows the laws of basic physics. A body in motion stays in motion unless acted on by an outside force. Your bike wants to roll forward. The more momentum it has, the more easily it does so. You are far more stable over small rocks and roots if you're carrying a little speed (because you have more momentum) than if you're crawling along getting bumped off course by every little obstacle in the path.

USE THE FORCE. That same fast, easy pedaling cadence that you use to speed down the road may send you nowhere fast on the trail. Though you should still aim for a comfortable, efficient cadence, you'll want to use a slightly lower gear and slower cadence to power through (rather than spin out on) difficult terrain.

RELAX. The first time you hit bumpy terrain, your initial instinct will be to tense up and hold on for dear life. But holding on too tight is counterproductive because it doesn't allow the bike to flow through the rocks and roots. Relax and keep your elbows and knees slightly bent at all times, so the bike has room to move beneath you as you gently guide it down the trail.

OR TAKE YOUR ROAD BIKE OFF ROAD. As their name implies, road bikes are designed to be ridden on, well, roads. But who says roads have to be paved? Some of my most memorable and enjoyable "road rides" have been where the pavement ends and turns to dirt, gravel, and cobbles. Try it yourself; you'll be pleasantly surprised where it takes you.

Of course, as you might expect, taking your road bike off road can be a little challenging. These tips can smooth the ride:

Hold on loosely. It's not just an old 38 Special love song; it's good dirt-riding advice as well. You want the bike to be free to move and soak up the bumps. If you're white-knuckling the bars and holding a lot of tension in your arms, the chattery bumps will feel bigger than they actually are, and you'll tire out sooner. Stay supple, with bent elbows, loose arms, and a light but firm grip on the bars.

Use the drops. When the road gets extra-rough, get down in the drops to lower your center of gravity, balance your weight, and have more control. Keep your shoulders relaxed and down.

Pack extra fuel. You use more muscles (and energy) riding off road, so you burn more calories. If you're going to be hitting lots of rough terrain, pack extra food.

RIDING IN THE RAIN

Even if you never start a ride in the rain, ride long enough and eventually you'll finish one in the wet, or at least get drizzled on along the way. Some cyclists actually enjoy riding in the rain. And for some who live in rainy climes, they embrace the rain because they'd never ride if they didn't. Whether you're a fair-weather rider or a duck on a bike, there are a few fundamentals you should know.

PROTECT YOUR CORE. Getting wet often means getting cold. If there's a chance of rain, pack a light jacket or at least a vest to keep your core warm. Your legs will be fine. But since your torso doesn't do much work and catches a lot of wind, it's the first thing to get cold. And when your core is cold, you're cold—and miserable.

AVOID SLIPPERY SURFACES. Manhole covers, storm grates, railroad tracks, and any other metal surfaces become slick as ice when wet. Avoid them. Road paint is also slippery when wet. Be alert for any rainbow slicks on

WHERE AM I?

Confession: I still can't do some of our most basic local rides without getting a little lost. I have absolutely no internal compass— none. I turn left when I should go right. I never know if I'm going east, west, south, or north (unless the sun is rising or setting, making it very obvious). This used to dissuade me from exploring. But then a funny thing happened: The more I explored, the less "lost" I became, because I soon saw how different roads intersected, and I became more familiar with the lay of the land. It's also easier than ever to find your way back from a steady string of wrong turns. Most smartphones have GPS apps that will at least let you pull up a map and show your bearing. Or, in the worst-case scenario, you can pull over and call someone who can help you out. If you're going to go exploring in less populated places, however, always take a friend (that's not a bad idea anytime). It's safer—and more fun—to get a little lost in good company.

the road, as well. They appear on patches of oil, and we don't have to tell you that oil is slick. Note, too, that the surface of the road itself will be most slick right as the rain begins because the moisture causes the oil that's settled into the pavement to rise to the surface.

BRAKE EARLY AND LIGHTLY. It takes longer to stop in the rain because your brakes first have to squeeze all the water from the rim before they can make contact to slow you down. You also don't want to brake too hard or suddenly because you're more likely to slide on slick roads. Squeeze your brakes lightly and steadily, well ahead of when you need to slow down or stop.

CORNER CAREFULLY. Usually when you corner, you lean the bike more than your body. When it's wet, you want to reverse that, so you keep as much tire contact with the pavement as possible. Shift weight to your outside pedal and keep your bike as upright as possible while leaning more with your body.

RELUBE THAT CHAIN LATER. Rain will wash away some of your chain lube, and your tires kick up dirt and grime that gets caught in your chain. Wash, dry, and lube your chain after riding in the rain.

TAKING A STAND

Getting in and out of the saddle is a skill that not only helps you tackle challenging, off-road, or rugged terrain as you advance in your cycling life, but also uses more muscles than seated riding, so it can help you improve your overall fitness.

The most natural time to use standing to your advantage is when you're climbing a particularly long and/or steep hill. It's also a useful maneuver when you want to get up to speed quickly, as making a quick dash across an intersection when the light turns yellow. Standing gives you an instant power boost by putting all your body weight into your pedals. The downside is that you also put more weight into your legs (especially if you have a larger upper body), which increases your overall workload. Because it's less efficient than seated pedaling, your heart rate goes higher, and you use about 10 percent more energy every time you stand.

So, it's wise to strike a balance and go with how you feel. If you have a relatively light upper body, you can probably stand more without feeling weighed down. If you're more muscular or heavier, staying seated longer will help you save energy. In any event, learning how to get in and out of the saddle is a skill that will help you tackle challenging terrain and give you a much-needed chance to stretch your legs on long rides. By practicing it, you can build your overall strength and fitness as well.

Here are a few tips for smooth standing.

SHIFT. Prepare for (and maximize) the burst of power you're going to get when you stand by shifting into a harder gear before getting out of the saddle. The exception: If you're standing because the hill is so steep you can barely turn the pedals anymore while seated, you obviously don't want to make it any harder. Just stay in the gear you're in.

STAND AS YOU GO OVER THE TOP. Stand smoothly as your lead foot comes over the top of the pedal stroke to maximize your power burst.

PUSH THE BIKE FORWARD. Be especially careful when standing when you are riding with a group. A common mistake riders make when they stand is inadvertently decelerating so their bike suddenly and dramatically slows right in front of the next rider, which can lead to that unfortunate rider colliding with their rear wheel and hitting the pavement. Shifting before you stand helps avoid this. Also, push your hands forward as you rise off the saddle to keep the bike directly beneath you as you stand.

LET IT SWAY. Leverage full power from the standing position by pulling up on the handlebars as you push into the pedals and allowing the bike to rock gently beneath you. You'll naturally lean forward a bit, but maintain your position in the center of the bike. The nose of the saddle should brush the backs of your legs.

PUSH AGAIN, AND SIT. When you're ready to sit, pedal evenly and push the bike forward again to put the bike right underneath you as you return to the saddle.

THE WORKOUT: UP AND AT IT

// **SKILL DRILL:** While pedaling smoothly, practice standing and sitting six to eight times, shifting gears to make the transition as seamless as possible. You can do this in a parking lot, on an empty stretch of road, or (ideally) up a small incline.

THE BYBO RIDE

TERRAIN: Undulating, preferably with a moderate hill

WHAT TO DO	INTENSITY	HOW LONG
Warmup	ZONE 1–2	~5 min
Pedal briskly	ZONE 2	15 min
Shift and stand	ZONE 2–3	30–60 sec
Sit and pedal	ZONE 2	2 min

Repeat this standing-and-sitting sequence 6 times (if you can do it on some inclines, even better)

Pedal briskly	ZONE 2	15 min

Finish at the pace of your choice going home.

TOTAL TIME: ~45–50 min

Perform this workout 3 times this week.

NOTE: *If you're already riding for longer than 50 minutes, simply extend the beginning or end of your ride or add another interval sequence.*

TAKE HOME: As mentioned earlier, you'll notice that you're working harder when you get up out of the saddle. Standing gives your legs a break and helps you get up steep hills because you're putting all your body weight into your pedals. But it raises your heart rate because your upper body has to work harder to support your torso and keep you balanced. This workout will help boost your fitness as well as your riding skills.

THE INSIDE RIDE

Similar to last week, this workout incorporates cardioresistance training, which blends cardio and strength training into the same workout. Once again, we'll mimic the outdoor ride and concentrate on getting in and out of the saddle to build fitness.

WHAT TO DO	INTENSITY	HOW LONG
Warmup	ZONE 1–2	~2–3 min
Steady, brisk, moderate resistance	ZONE 2	10 min
Increase resistance to simulate a moderate hill; stay smooth	ZONE 2–3*	2 min
Pick up your pace	ZONE 3	2 min
Increase resistance a bit and stand, picking up the pace as though cresting a climb	ZONE 3	30–60 sec
Sit back down, lower resistance, ease off the effort	ZONE 2 to 1	2 min

Dismount and perform the BYBO Core Workout.

Get back on the bike, spin for 2–3 min, and repeat the hill climb sequence once more (but do just one circuit of the Core Workout this time).

Finish with some easy stretching after you're done with the core moves.

TOTAL TIME: 45–50 min

This effort should feel like it's on the breaking point between aerobic and hard.

WEEK 6

WORKOUT LOG

Please log your workouts for the week.

WEEK 6				
BYBO Rides (including pleasure cruise) and Core Workout	Date: Notes:	Date: Notes:	Date: Notes:	Date: Notes:
Cross-training and/or rest	Date: Activity: Duration:	Date: Activity: Duration:	Date: Activity: Duration:	Date: Activity: Duration:

ANY OBSTACLES? _____

ACCOMPLISHMENTS? _____

OTHER NOTES. _____

BYBO CORE WORKOUT
(SEE PAGE 24 FOR EXERCISE DIRECTIONS)

Do the moves one after another like a circuit. Then repeat.

* Crank Plank
* Spiderman Pushup

* Figure 4 Bridge
* Tipping Bird

BYBO STRETCHES
(SEE PAGE 36 FOR STRETCH DIRECTIONS)

* Figure 4
* Stork
* Windshield Wiper

* Cobra
* Prayer Pose

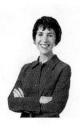

LESLIE'S LESSONS

BIKE YOUR BUTT OFF!
EATING PLAN: EAT TO RIDE (AGAIN)

Week 6 already! Wow, time flies when you are biking your butt off. And by now, 6 weeks in, I think you have made some discoveries about food, eating habits, and what feels good when you ride. Last week, we focused on health saboteurs, eating for and during your rides, and hydration. Now we are going to focus on recovery: what to eat after rides to ensure that your muscles heal properly so you can continue to make progress.

Let's talk recovery. What exactly does it mean? It is the time to restore, restock, rehydrate, and refuel so you can get out there and ride again without undue soreness or fatigue. New riders (and even not-so-new riders) make these common mistakes when it comes to recovery.

* Wait too long to refuel
* Eat too much or too little postride
* Drink too much or too little postride

* Wait too long to rehydrate
* Drink alcohol before rehydrating and refueling

Now we'll do it a better way. First of all, the goal is to eat *or* drink something containing calories within 15 to 30 minutes of finishing a ride. As is the case with prefueling, we are not talking about eating after an easy spin. You don't need to do any special recovery after easy rides. But certainly after a good, hard workout, you need to start the recovery process. The enzymes in the muscles that help with restocking the glycogen (stored carbohydrates) and also those that aid in protein synthesis and muscle repair are most active in the window immediately after exercise. Or, put another way, the longer you wait to refuel, the longer it takes your body to recover.

Here's what you need after a hard or long ride.

FLUIDS. Aim for 24 ounces of fluid for every pound you have lost. This doesn't need to be consumed within that 15- to 30-minute window, but rather over the duration of the day. For example, if you lost 2 pounds during your ride, you would need to consume 48 ounces of liquid over the rest of the day to bring your body back to optimal hydration.

CARB–PROTEIN MIX. You can get this from fluid or food. I suggest about 200 calories, such as what you'd get from the following:

- 10 ounces low-fat chocolate milk
- Gatorade Recover
- 8 ounces Odwalla or Naked smoothie
- A bar such as Kashi, Nature Valley, Lärabar, Luna
- Half a peanut butter and jelly sandwich
- ⅓ cup trail mix

Have only *one* of these items. It is a postexercise snack, not a postexercise meal. So have something with you that you can access quickly. If you really don't want to chew, you can refuel with a beverage, but it must have some protein. That is why I like milk or a smoothie, or a sports beverage with protein.

For those of you who say, "I am trying to lose weight and just burned some calories riding, why would I want to eat anything?," here is why. If you don't, you may be more likely to overeat later in the day. Make your postride fueling part of your cooldown.

On the flip side, for those of you that say, "Hey I rode for an hour, so I will finish my ride at Starbucks and chow down on a Mocha Frappuccino and a scone the size of my helmet," *don't even think about it*! The goal is to expend more calories than you take in, and you would have to have ridden for hours to burn all the calories in those foods.

In general, my motto after exercise is "Less is more." You don't need to eat a lot, but go two for two: both protein and some carbs. Let this chart be your guide.

INSTEAD OF	CHOOSE
Cereal bar	Bar with protein
Pretzels	Trail mix with nuts
Fruit	Fruit and yogurt or fruit with nut butter
Juice	Low-fat flavored milk
Sports drink	Sports drink with protein

BEING A LEAN RIDING MACHINE

Protein is important not only for recovery, but also for satiety (feeling satisfied for longer by what you eat) and muscle maintenance, which also help with improving fitness and weight loss. To be a lean, mean (okay, maybe not so mean) cycling machine, you should be consuming some protein as part of every meal. If you are comfortable with your current weight, choose the Maintain Plate; if you are looking to lose weight choose the Wane Plate.

Maintain Plate

- PROTEIN
- GRAINS
- FRUITS/VEGS

Wane Plate

- PROTEIN
- GRAINS
- FRUITS/VEGS

If you're tired of the same chicken breast, by all means expand your palate—and your plate. Try some of these excellent protein sources.

ANIMAL PROTEINS

- Extra-lean or ultra-lean ground beef
- Pork loin or chop
- Veal
- Lamb leg or loin
- Skinless poultry
- Ground turkey breast
- Fish
- Shellfish
- Low-fat milk
- Low-fat cottage cheese
- Reduced-fat cheese
- Eggs
- Greek yogurt

PLANT PROTEINS

- Tofu
- Soy milk
- Edamame
- Veggie burgers
- Beans such as kidney, black, chickpeas, navy
- Peas
- Nuts
- Nut butter
- Vegetables
- Grains
- Seeds

The only foods that do not contain protein are fruits, sweets, and oil. So if you have a turkey sandwich with vegetables on whole grain bread, you get protein from the turkey, veggies, and bread. A trifecta!

Protein foods require more calories for the body to digest. They help the body maintain lean mass, and they make you feel fuller for longer—all good reasons to include protein as part of every meal. But the secret is to pick lean protein, so no need for prime rib or fried shrimp!

How much protein do you need? A minimum of 0.5 grams per pound of body weight up to 0.9 grams per pound body weight. For those of you who use protein powders or bars, the protein in these products is part of your total for the day, not in addition to the protein you get in food.

To figure out what you need, use the following formula:

Desired weight × 0.5 = minimum number of grams of protein per day

And if you are trying to lose more:

Desired weight × 0.9 = number of grams of protein you need daily

Do your best to divide the protein as evenly as you can throughout the day. So don't have a day where you have minimal protein at breakfast and lunch and then sit down to a cow at dinnertime.

FEND OFF INFLAMMATION

The final part of the recovery picture both day to day and long-term is keeping inflammation at bay. Hard workouts result in a small amount of damage to your muscles, which then get stronger by healing. This process causes some inflammation—and hence soreness. Your body creates its own inflammation fighters when you exercise, but you can help it along with a healthy anti-inflammatory diet—because to train in pain sends exercise down the drain.

Now is a good time to incorporate some anti-inflammatory foods into your daily food plan. Likewise, there are foods that actually can create inflammation in your body. You'll want to eat less of them. Here is a guide to what to increase and decrease on your plate.

As a side note, increasing anti-inflammatory foods while decreasing inflammation-promoting foods will not only help you recover from hard workouts and ride better, it also has been shown to protect against heart disease, diabetes, cancer, and other common diseases.

INCREASE THESE ANTI-INFLAMMATORIES

- Fatty fish: salmon, halibut, sardines
- Green leafy vegetables
- Deep-orange veggies such as carrots, sweet potatoes, squash
- Extra-virgin olive oil (small amounts)
- Green tea

- Tart cherry juice
- Ginger—really, it helps
- Turmeric, a spice that contains curcumin, which is an anti-inflammatory
- Beans and lentils
- Cayenne and chile pepper—capsaicin is the active ingredient

Remember, these foods are not to be eaten in addition to less-healthy fare, but in the place of it. If you use olive oil, then don't use butter, or have salmon instead of chicken, or sweet potatoes instead of pasta.

Ginger is great for adding some zing to vegetables, a stir-fry, or even a smoothie—think pineapple–mango–ginger. You can keep fresh ginger in the freezer and grate as needed, or buy a tube of chopped ginger. Gourmet Garden makes one that is sold in the produce section. Stir a little into a squash soup and top the soup with a sprinkle of cinnamon. Delicious!

MINIMIZE THESE PRO-INFLAMMATORY FOODS

- Added sugars (read the labels; sugar shouldn't be at the top)
- Trans fats in stick margarines, baked goods, doughnuts, fried foods

- Saturated fats in poultry skin, butter, whole milk, full-fat cheese, regular ground beef, fatty meats, bacon, sausage

FOR THIS WEEK

EAT FOR RECOVERY. Be sure it's enough but not too much (about 200 calories), at the right time (15 to 30 minutes after exercise), and in the right balance (carbs and protein).

MUSCLE UP THE PLATE. Include protein in every meal.

REDUCE PAIN WHEN YOU TRAIN. Aim to consume anti-inflammatory foods daily.

Secrets of Their Success

CRYSTAL REESE, 34

WEIGHT LOST:
10 pounds, plus 3 inches off her waist

RUSSELL REESE, 36

WEIGHT LOST:
7 pounds, plus 2 inches off his waist

Crystal and Russ were like so many well-intentioned folks I meet. They enjoyed being active and knew they should be active, but, well, life and their jobs (his requires a fair amount of travel) often got in the way. So though they belonged to a gym, they didn't get there as often as they'd liked to. They were very excited to participate in the BYBO program as a way to kick themselves into gear.

"We have bikes and would like to get in the habit of riding them," Crystal told us early on. "We also belong to a gym that has Spin bikes, although neither of us has ever used them." Russ and Crystal are one of those couples who are genuinely best friends as well as husband and wife. They both were eager to learn some new fitness skills they could use together for life.

The first message we got from them was encouraging—and heartwarming. "Just wanted to tell you Russ and I are really enjoying ourselves. It's nice to 'have to' spend time together. :)" And for anyone who's ever wondered what a difference having a workout partner can make, Crystal's next message was equally heartwarming, if in a different way: "Our schedules have been all over the map and we have really been out of sync, as you will be able to tell

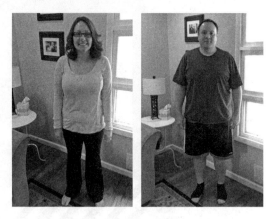

from our workout logs. I must say that having Russ in this 12-week ride has been an encouragement for me. I feel bad for people who do not have the encouragement of their partner."

Even when their workouts together "limped along," in Crystal's words, due to illness, travel snafus, or general fatigue, they kept each other going. And they kept making steady progress as a result. "I have managed to maintain a 10-pound weight loss, which for me is huge," Crystal noted. "Usually as soon as my main workouts start slipping, I start to gain weight. But I've taken advantage of the hotel gyms while we're traveling and have been staying active otherwise."

On the food side, both have really benefited from logging their food intake for the first few weeks. Russ, like many of us, chose too many foods from the starch category—rice, potatoes, and pasta. Through the BYBO plan, he learned to create a more balanced plate, one that included more fiber-rich foods and protein at every meal so he could feel satisfied longer. Leslie told him to go ahead and keep his favorite pasta dinners, but to dial back the size of the pasta serving and add shrimp, chicken, or meat sauce to improve the satiety. Russ, who typically ate more than half of his daily calories from dinner to bedtime, also benefited from making a shift in his eating patterns to better fuel up early on.

Crystal benefited from small tweaks to her diet. Swapping veggies for pita chips when she wanted something to pair with hummus dip, making her oatmeal with milk, and adding more protein to snacks and meals kept her diet more balanced and ultimately more satisfying. She was also mindful to eat only when she was hungry rather than mindlessly munching.

In the end, they were both thrilled with the results. They learned how to get a workout on their bikes and new skills for riding both inside and outside, as well as how to eat more healthfully on the road and at home. "It was a great opportunity to learn eating and exercise habits that we could fit into our life," says Crystal.

CHAPTER 7

PEDAL
WITH
PURPOSE

FOR BICYCLING ENTHUSIASTS, the pleasure of pedaling a bike is all the reason they need to go out and ride. But even die-hard cyclists often apply their pedal strokes to charity events, set goals, and sometimes even sign up for races to add to the fun and fuel their motivation to ride when they're busy, the weather isn't great, or they'd otherwise be inclined to bail on their bike for any number of reasons.

This week I encourage you to explore the wonderful world of BikeReg.com—an enormous portal to cycling-related events of all types. Just click on the tab for Recreational Rides and select your region, and voilà, you'll find shop rides (regularly scheduled rides that depart from a bicycle shop), charity rides, even organized workouts. Another good source of information is your local bike shop. Ask about bike clubs in your region. I belong to several in my area—both road and mountain bike—that hold their own organized rides throughout the year. Also keep an eye out for ride fliers and brochures at your local bike shop. Those tend to advertise easily accessible events right in your backyard.

Once you've perused the options, find an event that sounds like fun and sign up! You don't need to shoot for a century (100-mile ride) if you're just starting out, of course. Many organized rides offer a variety of distances to choose from, including 10- to 20-mile routes that are very beginner friendly. Just signing up and putting the event on your calendar will give you something to work toward and also provide the opportunity to meet other local riders like yourself. Choosing a charity that is close to your heart also puts that much more purpose into every pedal stroke.

SET SOME GOALS

Signing up for an event makes it easier to set riding goals. But even if you don't sign up for an organized ride, you should still set some goals. I know, I know. You *do* have goals. You want to get fit and maybe lose some weight and ride better. But sometimes those types of fuzzy goals aren't enough. Why? Because chances are, you'll never get there. What does "get fit" mean? Will the desire to lose those extra pounds long-term keep you on track in the short term? What do you want to ride better for? The more specific you can be—both in the immediate future and down the road—the more likely it is you'll stay on track.

Take some time to think about what motivated you to pick up this book in the first place. If the motivation was weight loss, go to page 51 in Chapter 2, do the calculations under Shed the Spare Tire, and set realistic weight-loss goals using the figures you come up with based on your body type. Losing more than $\frac{1}{2}$ pound to 2 pounds a week is unsustainable. Our most successful panelists over the long-term, like Carol Malazita (who whittled a full 4 inches off her waist), were the ones who kept chipping away slowly as their muscles firmed and fat burned off. At the end of the plan, they were a size smaller without feeling like they had undergone unreasonable challenges for 12 weeks. That's the goal.

Did you see yourself becoming a more capable cyclist? Set concrete stepping-stone goals that will take you there. Set a goal to be able to get a drink without having to stop to pull out your water bottle. Aim to ride a straight line while scanning over your shoulder for traffic. Set a destination goal, such as being able to ride to the coffee shop in the next town (and back, of course) or to complete a popular route in your area.

HEAD TO THE HILLS

As you expand your horizons as a cyclist, setting goals, planning adventures, and conquering charity rides, you're going to encounter some larger obstacles—hills, maybe even mountains. There are riders—even sage, seasoned

(continued on page 148)

CLIMBING THE CYCLING LADDER

New riders often struggle with goal setting because they don't have enough experience to know what they're capable of. This book is designed to make you a competent and confident cyclist over a 12-week span. This chart will help you as you progress to bigger and better rides.

If you've done COFFEE SHOP TRIPS, you're ready for:

COMMUTING. If you've negotiated the traffic to sip a soy latte at your local bean brewery, you're ready to saddle up for some more purposeful pedaling. A study by New York City's Transportation Alternatives shows that trips of less than 3 miles are often faster by bike than by car and that those 5 to 7 miles in length take about the same time as in an automobile and add up to 1,300 bonus miles a year! "Test different routes on the weekend to find a fun, scenic, or low-traffic route that you'll look forward to riding every day," suggests Carolyn Szczepanski, communications director at the League of American Cyclists. Oh, and use a rubber band to keep your pant leg out of your chain.

If you've done LONG WEEKEND RIDES, you're ready for:

SHOP AND/OR GROUP RIDES. Riding 2 to 3 hours with the right group is way easier than doing it on your own because you share the work and get a break from the wind. You learned the basics of pacelining in Chapter 5. Put them to use on a shop or group ride soon.

If you've done SHOP AND/OR GROUP RIDES OF ~3 HOURS, you're ready for:

METRIC CENTURY, CENTURY, AND/OR CHARITY RIDES. Group rides prepare you for the next step in natural cycling evolution—the charity ride, especially the coveted century (100-mile) ride. You can find rides near you on Web sites like BikeReg.com and Active.com and, of course, at your local bike shop. Give yourself at least 12 weeks to train (double that if you're relatively new to the sport). Increase your total riding time or mileage by about 10 percent week by week leading up to the event. Aim to hit a long ride of about 70 to 75 miles (about 5 hours of riding time) before the event. Definitely practice eating and drinking during your long rides. Taking in about 200 to 300 calories per hour—try fig bars, bananas, energy bars, and sports drink—will help you get to the finish line strong without bonking.

If you've done **CENTURIES**, you're ready for:

MS 150 OR OTHER 2- TO 3-DAY RIDES OR TOURS. Your first thought after completing a 100-mile ride may not be "Hey, I'd like to do that again tomorrow." But multiday rides are easier than you think, not to mention fun and rewarding. Primarily you need to condition your body so you will be comfortable with consecutive long days on the bike. Perform your century training as normal and gradually increase your Sunday ride mileage (assuming your long-ride day is Saturday) to about half the goal distance. "Postride recovery also becomes paramount," says Andy Applegate, who coaches many riders through multiday affairs. "The next-day recovery starts on day one. Eat enough so you don't finish depleted. Then stock your glycogen stores ASAP and elevate those legs when you're done, so you're ready for the next day."

If you've done **MS 150 RIDES**, you're ready for:

A BIKE ADVENTURE! There are countless multiday tours across the country—and the world—through organizations like Backroads and Trek Travel. Or try your hand at one of the beginner-friendly multiday charity rides like the Arthritis Foundation's California Coast Classic. Sure, these rides are long, but they're well supported, usually travel through gorgeous locations, and you're pedaling for a good cause.

ones—who will pedal miles out of their way to avoid these vertical challenges. I say embrace them. They're a surefire way to become stronger, and there is nothing as satisfying as cresting the top of a long, tough climb ... except maybe going down the other side (but more on that in a bit).

Pedaling against the force of gravity builds strength in your legs, improves your cardiovascular fitness, scorches calories, and greatly increases your confidence. Yes, hills are hard. But you don't have to hate them. Here's how to crest even the steepest climbs with confidence.

CONQUER ANY CLIMB—WITH A SMILE

Many moons ago, I was at one of my first big races in West Virginia, which they don't call the mountain state for nothing. I was at the foot of the biggest climb—a 2-mile monster that I was dreading to my bones. I put my head down and pedaled by another rider fixing his bike roadside. He looked up at me with the easiest smile I'd ever seen and very sweetly and sincerely said, "Hey, enjoy the climb."

Huh? "Enjoy the climb?" Was he high? (Actually he could've been given the location, but that's a different story.) I raised my chin to look up at the hill before me and thought, "You know? Why not try?" Immediately, my shoulders relaxed. The death grip I had on my handlebars loosened. I felt a little lighter. I smiled. The hill was just as long and just as steep as it had been before, but this time up it felt easier because I decided to embrace it in a positive fashion rather than just put my head down and suffer my way to the top. I've taken the same approach with every hill ever since. You can too. Here's how.

RELAX. Many riders tense up at the mere sight (or thought!) of a climb, gripping the handlebars hard, tensing up their forearms, shoulders, and even faces. All that tension wastes valuable energy that could be propelling you up the hill. As you approach the hill, start releasing the tension in your head and relax your face, shoulders, arms, and hands. Wiggle your fingers while loosely gripping the bars. This is how you should feel when you're climbing.

BRACE YOUR CORE. Your torso provides the platform that your legs press off from as you pedal up a hill. As you gently pull back on the bars, your core body muscles also transfer power from your upper body to your lower body pushing into the pedals. You want that core to be solid (hence the core exercises you've been doing). Consciously keep it a bit taut while you climb. Pulling in your elbows so they're closer to your torso can help.

SIT AND SPIN. Remember, every time you get out of the saddle, your heart rate gets higher as you use more energy to support your body weight. Sitting and spinning in a relatively easy gear is the most efficient way to get up a hill. That doesn't mean you have to stay stuck in one position as if you're glued to the saddle. In fact, you can recruit different muscles by moving around. For gradual grades, scoot your butt back and sit rearward on the saddle. Shift up toward the nose when the going gets steep, and gently pull the bars to assist you up the hill.

SHIFT AND STAND. For long climbs you'll want to stand occasionally to stretch your legs. For steep climbs, you'll want to stand to leverage your body weight to propel the bike up the incline. This is where the standing drills from last week come in handy. Just click into the next-hardest gear (unless you're on a really steep incline and need to stand to just keep moving forward!) before you stand to maintain your momentum when you get out of the saddle. Remember to push the bike forward a bit so it stays underneath you as you stand. After a few pedal strokes, shift into an easier gear and sit back down.

BREATHE DEEP AND STEADY. You want to climb right below what is known as your lactate threshold—a fancy way of saying the point at which your legs start burning and your muscles want to shut down. The easiest way to manage your pace is by paying attention to your breathing. It's natural to breathe heavily up a climb. But once you go from smooth but labored breathing to panting, you've crossed the line into blowup territory. Slow down until your breathing is back in control.

ROLL OUT LIKE A CARPET. Riders often mistakenly charge too hard at the beginning of a climb, only to fade like an old pair of blue jeans halfway to the top. Instead, start a little bit slower and easier and ratchet up your speed as you work your way to the top. Think of your pace like a carpet unrolling, picking up speed and momentum as it goes. Your goal is to finish the climb more briskly than you began it. It often helps to stand and give a few strong pedal strokes right as you come to the crest to kick you over the top.

WHAT GOES UP . . .

What goes up must come down, of course. For some cyclists, descending is exhilarating. Others find it slightly (or in some cases completely) terrifying. I'd be remiss if I told you how to get to the top of a climb without providing some advice for getting down the other side. The following tips will make you a more confident descender. (Start with a short, straight downhill you can descend without hitting the brakes and practice getting in the correct position.)

GET BACK, DIP LOW. If descents make you nervous, your first instinct might be to sit bolt upright to slow yourself down. Doing so actually makes you more unstable and less safe because your weight is too high and too far forward. Instead, shift your rear back, spreading your weight over the bicycle, and put your hands on the drops on a road bike, or simply bend your arms and lower your torso if you're riding with flat bars. This lowers your center of gravity, keeps the rear wheel firmly on the ground, and makes the bike handle more predictably.

EASY ON THOSE BRAKES. Yes, I know you want to grab fistfuls of brakes and squeeze with all your might when the speed gets scary. But resist the urge! Instead, feather your brakes (i.e., lightly squeeze them on and off) to scrub speed and keep your descent controlled and comfortable. Remember, your front (left) brake possesses the lion's share of your stopping power, so go easy on it. Remember what you practiced in Week 1.

USE YOUR CORNERING SKILLS. There are often twists and turns on descents, which is why we practiced cornering early on. The same rules apply when you're taking turns in a descent. You want to brake as much as you can *before* the turn, because when you brake, your bike stands up and goes straight—the opposite of what you want in a turn. Remember to lean your bike (not your body). Press your outside foot into that pedal. Point the other knee to the inside of the turn to shift your hips and shoulders into the turn. Look where you want the bike to go. It will follow your head and eyes. Make the turn as "straight" as possible by starting wide (without crossing the yellow line), cutting through the apex, and exiting wide.

WORKOUT: UP, UP, AND AWAY!

// SKILL DRILL: *Relax!*

Starting at the top of your head, progressively relax your body. Relax your forehead, eyes, cheeks, mouth, jaws, neck, shoulders, chest, back, arms, and hands. Wiggle your fingers. Position yourself for maximum oxygen consumption. Keep your back straight and chest open. Take note of how you feel. This is how you want to feel before any hill (or hill effort if you're on the trainer).

THE BYBO RIDE

TERRAIN: Rolling to hilly

WHAT TO DO	INTENSITY	HOW LONG
Warmup	ZONE 1–2	15 min
On a moderate climb, shift into a gear that allows you to pedal at a cadence of about 80 rpm (steep hills may require a slower cadence); pedal seated	ZONE 2–3	2–3 min
Shift, stand, and pedal	ZONE 3	30 sec
Coast back down the climb and pedal easy	ZONE 1–2	2–3 min
Repeat the climbing sequence 2 more times*		
Ride at a brisk cadence	ZONE 2	10 min

Finish with easy pedaling going home.

TOTAL TIME: ~45 min

Perform this workout 3 times this week.

This is a classic "hill repeat" workout. This type of workout is excellent for building fitness but is not everybody's cup of tea. If you have a convenient hill, I suggest you give it a try. You also can ride a hilly route and do the climbing drill on two or three hills along the way.

NOTE: *If you're already riding for longer than 45 minutes, simply extend the beginning or end of your ride or add another interval sequence.*

TAKE HOME: Hill workouts can be taxing if you're unaccustomed to inclines. If you find yourself tired and a bit sore from the effort, swap one BYBO workout for one flat, easy spin of the same duration.

THE INSIDE RIDE

As in previous weeks, this workout incorporates cardioresistance training, which blends cardio and strength training in the same workout. Once again, we'll mimic the outdoor ride and concentrate on hill climbing (get ready to crank that resistance), which is one of the best ways to build fitness and strength fast.

WHAT TO DO	INTENSITY	HOW LONG
Warmup	ZONE 1–2	10 min
Increase resistance to simulate a moderate climb that allows you to pedal at a cadence of about 80 rpm; pedal seated	ZONE 2–3	2–3 min
Increase resistance, stand, and pedal	ZONE 3	30 sec
Sit and decrease the resistance to easy	ZONE 1–2	2–3 min
Repeat the climbing sequence once more		
Pedal at your normal speed, easing off for the final 30 sec	ZONE 2–1	~1 min
Dismount and perform the BYBO Core Workout		
Get back on the bike, spin for ~2 min, and repeat the hill climb sequence (do just one circuit of the Core Workout this time)		
Pedal easy to cool down	ZONE 2–1	~3–5 min

Finish with some easy stretching once you're done.
TOTAL TIME: ~45 min

WORKOUT LOG

Please log your workouts for the week.

WEEK 7				
BYBO Rides (including pleasure cruise) and Core Workouts	Date: Notes:	Date: Notes:	Date: Notes:	Date: Notes:
Cross-training and/or rest	Date: Activity: Duration:	Date: Activity: Duration:	Date: Activity: Duration:	Date: Activity: Duration:

ANY OBSTACLES? _____

ACCOMPLISHMENTS? _____

OTHER NOTES: _____

BYBO CORE WORKOUT
(SEE PAGE 24 FOR EXERCISE DIRECTIONS)

Do the moves one after another like a circuit. Then repeat.

* Crank Plank
* Spiderman Pushup

* Figure 4 Bridge
* Tipping Bird

BYBO STRETCHES
(SEE PAGE 36 FOR EXERCISE STRETCH DIRECTIONS)

* Figure 4
* Stork
* Windshield Wiper

* Cobra
* Prayer Pose

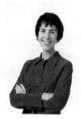

LESLIE'S LESSONS

BIKE YOUR BUTT OFF! EATING PLAN: MOVING FORWARD, EATING SMARTER

Six weeks done. You've been biking, eating, writing, and making lifestyle changes on every front. You've accomplished much thus far, and there's plenty more to go! So before we move forward to the second half of the plan, I want you to think about the past 6 weeks from an eating perspective.

What have you changed, tweaked, or modified in the following categories?

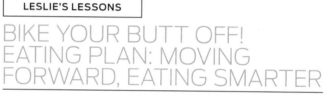

EATING HABITS

* Number of meals?
* Rate of eating?

* Meal locations?

FOOD CHOICES

* Different variety?
* Portions?

* New foods?

* Drinking enough?

* Different choices?

* Drinking less soda, alcohol, sugary drinks?

Pre- and postride fuel and fluids?

What are you doing now that you've never done before?

How do you feel?

Oftentimes, when my clients are trying to "healthen up" their eating, they tend to restrict the amounts they eat and their food choices. Granted, correctly sized portions are essential for weight loss and maintenance, but if your circle of foods is too small, you will get bored and be more easily tempted by indulgent items.

So here are some suggestions to expand your food horizons.

SPICE UP YOUR MEALS

* Dress up that same old chicken dish by slathering on a curry-yogurt sauce or sautéing the chicken in olive oil with a little bit of a chile pepper.

* Add chopped mango to salsa and serve over fish.

* Try a blackened seasoning rub on flank steak.

INSTEAD OF STEAMED VEGGIES, TRY

* Roasted vegetables: Chop zucchini, bell peppers, mushrooms, onions, carrots, and place on a cookie sheet sprayed with cooking spray. Drizzle on a little olive oil, and add herbs to taste. Roast at 450°F for 10 to 15 min.

* Stir-fried vegetables

* Grilled vegetables

* Pureed vegetables served as a soup

WHAT ABOUT GRAINS?

* Brown rice *again*? Of course you're bored! Try adding some chopped dried plums and toasted almonds.

* Try quinoa for a change of taste.

* Cook bulgur in chicken broth and add sautéed onions.

* For pasta: Try angel hair; the noodles are thinner, so it looks like more on your plate.

WEEK 7

EAT A VARIETY OF FATS

* Olive oil is wonderful, but try some variations such as lemon olive oil, or add some basil or garlic to the oil.

* Try guacamole to replace mayonnaise.

* Go nuts! Besides peanut butter, now you can find almond, hazelnut, and cashew butters.

* You can eat nuts plain or roast them or toast them, but do watch the amount. The calories add up quickly.

HOW ABOUT CHANGING WHAT IS IN YOUR GLASS OR MUG?

* Make spiced tea by adding a cinnamon stick or a little grated ginger.

* Add a splash of apple cider to tea.

* Try a cinnamon-flavored coffee or add a little cocoa powder.

* Try herbal teas for lots of flavor without the caffeine. How about buying a variety pack so you have lots of choices?

* Think soup as a liquid and also a food—squash bisque, a hearty tomato soup, or even bean soup.

HOW ABOUT SOME NEW GADGETS?

* Consider a kitchen scale so you really know how much you're eating.

* How about a grill pan to bring summer tastes to your indoor stove?

* A grater is good for grating ginger, garlic, and nutmeg to add more flavor to foods.

* A Misto oil sprayer allows you to add controlled quantities of oil.

* A microwave popcorn popper gives you the freedom to add the flavorings you want.

* A single-serve blender is great for mixing smoothies, pureeing vegetables, or making soups.

* I like collapsible measuring cups. Put one in your cereal box, oatmeal container, or jar of nuts as a visual reminder of the correct portion size.

And on the subject of spicing things up, try broadening your palate with the following.

SWEET SPICES	
Ginger	Allspice
Nutmeg	Anise
Clove	Fennel
Cinnamon	Cardamom

SAVORY SPICES	
Garlic powder	Coriander
Onion powder	Basil
Cayenne pepper	Tarragon
Dill	Oregano
	Rosemary

MIXED SPICES	
Chili powder	Curry powder

FOR GREAT TASTE	
Sea salt	Cracked black pepper

Many supermarkets offer small bags of spices and herbs. And many companies offer spice blends or grinders. Gourmet Garden makes tubes of herbs and spices that are sold in the produce aisle. You do need to refrigerate these products. In addition, maybe you can join a spice and herb co-op with a few friends. Each of you buys a few different items and then you share them—like a cookie exchange but with a lot fewer calories. You can be spice girls (or boys).

My assignment for you this week is to try something new.

- A different preparation method
- A different food
- An unfamiliar seasoning
- A new gadget

So, to keep the monotony away, let your taste buds stray. You will be surprised by how easily little tweaks translate into increased enjoyment and satisfaction, and weight-loss success!

CHAPTER 8

STRENGTHEN YOUR FRAME

(THE HUMAN ONE, THAT IS!)

OTHER THAN PERHAPS SWIMMING, there are few physical activities as gentle on your body as cycling. It's easy on your joints. You can make it as challenging or as relaxing as you'd like. You can coast (can't do that for very long in the water). Because the bike supports your weight, it's also easier for the average (and maybe overweight) person to sprint, tackle steep climbs, and otherwise put in hard efforts than it is with other forms of exercise, like running.

This week we'll focus on some of those hard efforts, particularly sprinting (don't worry if you haven't "sprinted" since third-grade recess; it's all relative), not only because it's fun but also because cranking up the intensity is good for the body as well as the soul. Sprinting is a form of high-intensity interval training (HIIT)—a fancy name for short bursts of hard effort. Numerous studies have shown that by incorporating some HIIT into your usual cardio routine, you can dramatically improve your cardiovascular fitness, increase fat loss, and improve overall health. A recent study published in *Medicine and Science in Sports and Exercise* showed that HIIT reduced blood pressure and improved glucose tolerance, while a similar study published in *Exercise and Sport Sciences Reviews* showed that HIIT delivers more heart benefits than regular cardio alone.

Because high-intensity efforts demand more work from your whole body, we'll also focus on proper recovery techniques, eating to build muscles and bones, and how to troubleshoot common aches and niggles like numb hands and achy knees that can come from improper technique and bike position.

NEED FOR SPEED

Lets face it: It's fun to go fast. Speed is exhilarating. Even riders who claim "I don't care about going fast" probably enjoy the rush that comes with the feeling of flying on a bike. How fast can you go? Top-notch sprinters can hit 40 miles per hour on the flats. The rest of us mere mortals can reach into the 20s and 30s with work. Speed work also improves your top-end fitness, which means that over time, your average riding speed will increase as well.

This week we'll tap into that inner speed demon and work on cranking up the miles per hour, at least for short stretches. Though your legs are doing the lion's share of the work when you pick up the pace, riding fast is very much a full-body affair. Here are some cues to keep in mind as you turn on your turbo.

KEEP YOUR UPPER BODY QUIET. Your upper body provides the platform for your legs to push off of, in essence counterbalancing the effort of your lower body. That means you want it to be rock solid and steady when you're going really fast. In Spin classes I'll tell people to pretend they have glasses of wine perched on their shoulders and they shouldn't spill a drop. Try to imagine the same as you're charging down the road.

FOCUS ON THE UPSWING. It's easy to let your pedal stroke fall apart when you're ramping up the revolutions per minute. Keep it controlled by focusing on the upstroke, driving those knees up toward the bars. This will keep you from mashing down on the pedals and losing your fluid, circular spin.

BELLY BREATHE. Sprinting is hard work, so you need plenty of oxygen. You also need to stay calm and controlled to maximize your efficiency. Focus on drawing deep belly breaths to deliver all the oxygen you can to your working muscles and to avoid the gasping and panting that come from taking shallow breaths.

WORKOUT: DEMON SPEED!

TERRAIN: Flat to undulating

// **SKILL DRILL:** Jump-Starts

"Jumping" out of the saddle is the best way to get up to speed quickly. To execute a jump, shift into a harder gear, stand up on the pedals, and take a few hard, fast pedal strokes out of the saddle to build your speed and cadence. Once you've got those pedals spinning at a brisk cadence, sit back down and continue pedaling at high speed while keeping your form smooth and in control, shifting as needed to keep your speed. It's best to be warmed up before you launch a full sprint. So practice these at about half speed to get the hang of jumping out of the saddle to pick up your pace. Practice 5 to 10 jump-starts in a parking lot or on an empty stretch of road.

THE BYBO RIDE

TERRAIN: Flat to undulating

WHAT TO DO	INTENSITY	HOW LONG
Warmup	ZONE 1–2	10 min
Increase pace/intensity	ZONE 2	15 min
Shift up to a harder gear and perform a jump-start. When you get up to speed, sit down and pedal as fast as you can (once you're in the saddle).	ZONE 4	30 sec
Lower the pace/intensity	ZONE 2	1–2 min

Repeat the jump-start/recover sequence 5 more times.

Finish with easy pedaling going home.

TOTAL TIME: ~50 min

Perform this workout 3 times this week.

TAKE HOME: There's a saying in cycling circles: The only way to get fast is to ride fast. Sounds obvious, but many riders neglect speed work and then lament that they aren't faster. These workouts will make you faster by training your muscles to push hard and by conditioning your body to better convert oxygen into energy.

NOTE: *If you're already riding for longer than 50 minutes, simply extend the beginning or end of your ride or add another interval sequence.*

THE INSIDE RIDE

This week, we're going to break away from the cardioresistance format and keep you on the bike for the full workout before hitting the floor for four new core moves. As in previous weeks, however, we'll mimic the outdoor ride and concentrate on high-speed, sprint-style riding, which improves your top-end fitness and is fun to do.

WHAT TO DO	INTENSITY	HOW LONG
Warmup	ZONE 1–2	10 min
Increase pace/intensity	ZONE 2	15 min
Increase resistance and perform a jump-start.* When you get up to speed, sit down and pedal as fast as you can (once in the saddle).	ZONE 4	30 sec
Lower the pace/intensity	ZONE 2	1–2 min
Repeat the jump-start/recover sequence 5 more times		
Ease back and cool down	ZONE 2 to 1	2–3 min

Perform the Core Workout.

Finish with some easy stretching after you're done.

TOTAL TIME: ~50 min

See the Jump-Starts Skill Drill in the BYBO workout on page 162; it's the same on an indoor bike, you're just stationary.

WORKOUT LOG

Please log your workouts for the week.

WEEK 8				
BYBO Rides (including pleasure cruise) and Core Workouts	Date: Notes:	Date: Notes:	Date: Notes:	Date: Notes:
Cross-training and/or rest	Date: Activity: Duration:	Date: Activity: Duration:	Date: Activity: Duration:	Date: Activity: Duration:

ANY OBSTACLES? _____

ACCOMPLISHMENTS? _____

OTHER NOTES: _____

BYBO CORE WORKOUT

(SEE PAGE 24 FOR EXERCISE DIRECTIONS)

Do the moves one after another like a circuit. Then repeat.

- Crank Plank
- Spiderman Pushup

- Figure 4 Bridge
- Tipping Bird

BYBO STRETCHES

(SEE PAGE 36 FOR EXERCISE STRETCH DIRECTIONS)

- Figure 4
- Stork
- Windshield Wiper

- Cobra
- Prayer Pose

MAKE A SPEEDY RECOVERY

Fresh legs are a bike rider's best friends. And I'll confess, after a few hard workouts, yours might feel more like frenemies. Following hard days with easy recovery days is one way to get in their good graces again, as is eating plenty of muscle-mending foods (which you'll find in this and other chapters). But to make your legs your BFFs (best friends forever, if you don't have texting kids), give them some TLC with these special recovery techniques.

SPIN THEM OUT AND PROP THEM UP

Cooling down after hard efforts with a few minutes of easy spinning helps promote recovery by flushing out your legs and preventing blood from pooling in them, which can happen when you come to a dead stop after a challenging ride. When you get back home, stretching out a bit and propping your legs up for about 10 minutes will also allow the blood in your large lower-body muscles to circulate back around your body, so you can get fresh oxygen and nutrients into those worked muscles and clear out the waste.

GIVE YOUR MUSCLES A SQUEEZE

During the past decade, compression wear—socks, tights, and shorts that are made of specially graded elastic material that promotes blood flow from your lower extremities back up to your heart—has grown from a small niche market used mostly by nurses and others who are on their feet all day to a staple in nearly every runner's, cyclist's, and triathlete's wardrobe. Do you need it? No. But you might love it—I know I do. Research suggests that compression tights help reduce blood lactate levels and speed recovery. Studies also show that athletes feel fresher and experience less muscle soreness after wearing them. I just know they make my legs feel fresh and happy. I swear by mine for long flights and have been known to even sleep in them on occasion.

The downside is cost. Compression doesn't come cheap. A set of full tights generally runs in the vicinity of $90 to $140 (though they last for years if properly cared for). If that's too much to chew, start with a pair of socks for just about $10. Popular brands include 2XU, SKINS, and Zoot.

ICE, ICE BABY

Marathoners and other endurance athletes swear by icy-cold water dunks postactivity to help clear lactic acid and reduce inflammation—and thereby soreness—following long, hard efforts. Studies that have examined how effective this practice is at clearing lactic acid have found mixed results, but most researchers agree that athletes feel less fatigued and sore after an ice bath and may even perform better during subsequent efforts. The trick is doing it.

During the summer, I've been known to wade into a cold stream or a swimming pool after a hard ride. But there's no way in a million hard rides that I can get myself to fill my bathtub with icy water and take a dip. That said, if I have a particularly achy spot, I'll definitely swaddle it in a cold wrap or treat it to a bag of frozen peas for 15 or 20 minutes—works every time.

KEEP ON ROLLING

Perhaps my favorite form of recovery is rolling along my foam roller. Foam rollers are cylinders made of pressed Styrofoam (or other material) that you can use for self-massage. Like a cable that's been crimped one too many times, your hardworking muscles eventually develop kinks—small adhesions or knots that make you stiff and sore, preventing you from pedaling with full, unhindered mobility and power.

"Rolling along these rollers provides myofascial release [breaks adhesions and scar tissue within the muscle and the fascia that covers the muscle], warms and stretches the muscles, and increases circulation," says Scott Levin, MD, sports medicine specialist at Somers Orthopaedic Surgery and Sports Medicine Group in Carmel, New York. "It's convenient and very effective, because it allows you to home in on your problem spots and work them to your comfort level. Done after a hard workout or ride, rolling also can prevent delayed onset muscle soreness," he says.

I've gotten to the point that as soon as I feel even the slightest twinge of pain along my iliotibial (IT) band (a long band of fibrous tissue that runs from your hips to your knees and can cause pain in both joints when it gets bound up), I reach for my roller and nip it in the bud.

As a cyclist, you can develop tight, knotted spots in your leg muscles, of course, but also in your back's, which support you during long, hard rides. You can hit 'em all with your roller. Follow these directions, slowly rolling back and forth over the targeted muscle group about 10 to 12 times. If a spot feels tender, hold the roller there and press your weight into it, then roll through it until it feels better. You can roll daily or even several times daily, but aim for at least two or three times a week to keep your muscles supple.

CALVES

Sit on the floor with your legs straight out, hands on the floor behind you supporting your weight. Place the roller under your knees. Slowly roll along the back of your legs, up and down from your knees to your ankles.

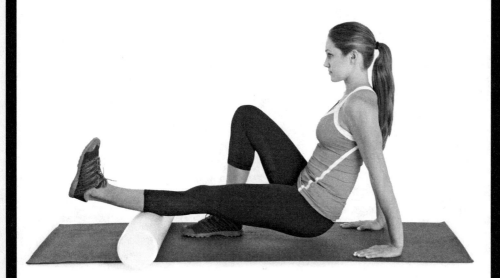

WEEK 8

HAMSTRINGS

Sit with your left leg on the roller; bend your right knee and put your hands on the floor behind you. Roll up and down from your knee to just under your left butt cheek. Switch legs.

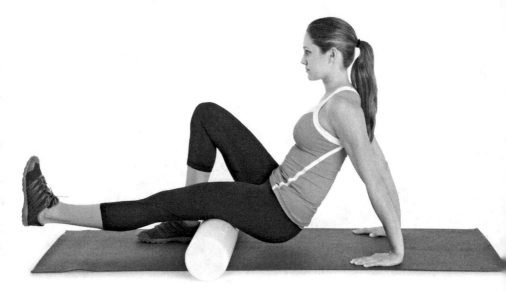

QUADS

Lie facedown on the floor and place the roller under your hips. Lean on your left leg and roll up and down from your hip to your knee. Switch legs.

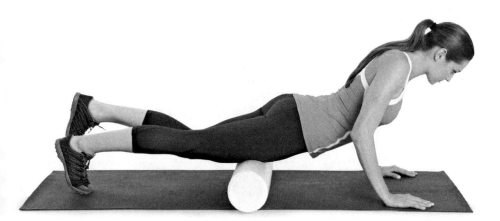

IT BAND

Lie on your side with the roller placed just below your hip. Bend your top leg and place that foot on the floor in front of your body for balance and to control the amount of pressure on the roller. Roll down along the outside of the leg from the hip to the knee and back up again. Switch legs.

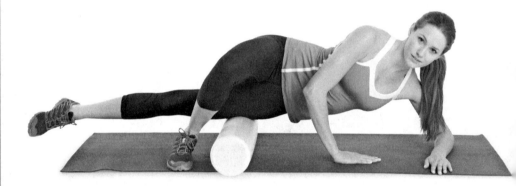

BUTT

Sitting on the foam roller, cross your left leg over your right knee and lean toward the left hip, putting your weight on your hands for support. Slowly roll one butt cheek over the roller. Switch sides.

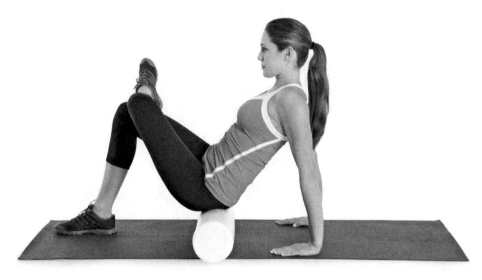

BACK

Sit on the floor with the foam roller behind you. Lace your fingers behind your head and lean your upper back onto the roller. Tighten your abs and glutes and slowly move up and down the roller.

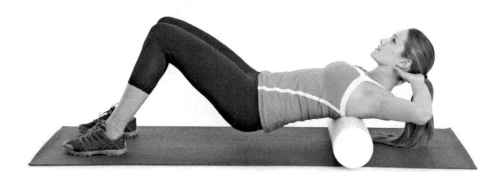

ADDUCTOR

Assume a plank position on the floor, supporting yourself on your toes and forearms. Bend your right leg and drape it over the roller, so it is parallel to your body with the roller resting against your groin muscles. Sink your weight into the roller and roll along the length of your inner thigh to your knee and back again. Switch sides.

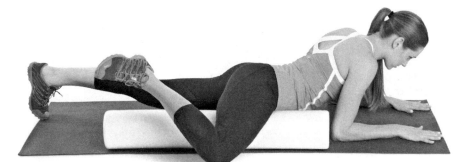

NO PAIN, ALL GAIN

As you begin racking up the miles, niggling aches and pains can start piping up. "With new riders the blame is usually poor bike fit or equipment setup or a training error, like going out for 50 miles on their first ride of the season," says Andy Pruitt, EdD, director of Boulder Center for Sports Medicine in Colorado and author of Andy Pruitt's Complete Medical Guide for Cyclists. *In seasoned cyclists, it's generally wear and tear in the form of "-itises," such as bursitis, or some degenerative joint diseases that can naturally occur over time, and you have to make a few changes to compensate, he says. This troubleshooting guide will help to quell—and correct—the most common nagging ouches before they become injuries. Sharp pain, however, is always a sign that something is wrong and you should see your doc.*

WHERE DOES IT HURT?	WHAT'S WRONG	THE FIX
FOOT	Hot spots, pain under the ball of your foot, and/or numb toes happen when pressure is concentrated on one small part of the sole of your foot and/or nerves are squeezed between your foot bones. Hot spots can happen to even longtime cyclists who've never had foot pain because the fat pads in our feet shrink over time, leaving the nerves in our feet less protected, says Pruitt.	For simple numbness, try loosening your shoes. Already loose? Opt for a wider shoe. For burning pain, slide your cleats all the way back; switch to shoes with a stiffer sole; try pedals with wider platforms.
ANKLE	Pain in the back of the ankle between the heel and calf is a symptom of Achilles tendonitis. It generally is brought on by doing too much (especially climbing) too soon. Having your cleats too far forward, which makes you pedal on your toes, can also strain the Achilles. "It's rarely just cycling, but generally also hiking and running, that causes Achilles problems," says Pruitt. "But you can ease on-the-bike pain with adjustments."	Rest, ice, and anti-inflammatories, so it doesn't become chronic. Move cleats back. Stretch by standing on a step with the ball of your foot on the step and the heel hanging off the edge. Drop the heel as far as possible. Hold 20 seconds. Switch legs. Build up mileage gradually.

WHERE DOES IT HURT?	WHAT'S WRONG	THE FIX
KNEE	"Cyclists' most common pain, and it hits all riders from paid pros to fitness enthusiasts in equal numbers," says Pruitt. "The knee is the victim, but the culprits are the hip above and the foot and ankle below." Incorrect saddle and/or cleat position, weak outer glutes, and doing too much too soon, especially in a big gear, can make your hinges hurt.	Get a professional bike fitting. As a rule of thumb, if it hurts in the front of your knee, your saddle is too low. Pain in the back of the knee means it's too high. Spin an easier gear. Strengthen your outer glutes with lateral leg exercises like side lunges and side leg raises. Stretch your quads, IT bands, and hamstrings regularly.
HIP	Pushing excessively high gears can wreak havoc on your hips, as can tight muscles and weak glutes.	Ride in easier gears and increase your cadence to take pressure off your hips. Follow the glute-strengthening advice (see Knee). Stretch your hips.
BACK	Often back pain can be blamed on simple fatigue and age-related wear and tear. Other common causes are poor bike fit and inadequate core strength.	Perform plank exercises to strengthen your core. Stretch your hamstrings. Check your bike fit to see that you're not "overreaching" (see Neck), keeping in mind that over the years you may need to tweak your position to accommodate changes in flexibility.
HAND	Numb, tingly fingers and/or painful wrists are generally caused by placing too much pressure on the nerves in your hand. You may have too much weight on your hands or have your wrists cocked at too extreme an angle.	Wear lightly padded gloves. Hold the bar with your wrists in a neutral position (like the position they're in when you shake hands). Check that the nose of your saddle isn't tipped down, shifting your weight too far forward and onto your hands.
NECK	Poor fit. Too much tension through shoulders and upper back.	The most common culprit is overreaching. When you look at the front wheel with your hands on the hoods, your bars should obstruct your hub. Keep your shoulders down and relaxed.

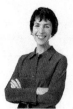

BIKE YOUR BUTT OFF! EATING PLAN: DRINK UP, EAT RIGHT, TRAIN BETTER, HURT LESS

We're 8 weeks in, and you've been riding more, riding harder, and feeling it. Bravo. Now is the time to make sure you are drinking enough, and at the right time and of the right fluids.

Why is this so important? First off, your body is made of approximately 60 percent water. You can lose between 2.5 and 3 liters—a large soda bottle's worth—of water every day, and that does not account for fluid losses with exercise. Proper hydration is very important because we need water for all our vital functions, including the following:

- To maintain the health of the cells
- For healthy circulation
- To get rid of waste
- To regulate body temperature

- To lubricate and cushion joints
- To aid with digestion
- To moisturize the skin
- To carry nutrients and oxygen to the cells

So let's take a closer look at what counts as a fluid and what the optimal choices are for being well hydrated as well as for losing weight.

BEST BETS	NOT SO HOT
Water	Soda (regular or diet)
Unsweetened or herbal tea	Sweet tea or bottled teas
Unsweetened coffee	Sweetened coffee beverages
Small glass of juice (6 ounces)	Large glass of juice
Skim milk	Whole milk
Low-fat milk	Milk shakes
Soy milk, light	Soy milk, full-fat
Sparkling water	Lemonade
Broth	Cream soup
Vegetable soup	Bisques made with cream
Tomato soup	Fruit punch and fruit drinks
Energy drinks	

You may have heard that caffeine dehydrates the body and therefore coffee, tea, and cola beverages do not count, but that is not true. You may find that you have to void more quickly after consuming a caffeinated beverage, but you will not dehydrate. The beverages in the Not So Hot column are there because they are higher in sugar and/or fat.

You might be thinking, "What about that beer after a ride or celebratory champagne after my first race?" Alcohol is the only beverage that *is* a diuretic. That doesn't mean you can't drink it, but it does not count toward your daily total. And the calorie cost can be high. What is a drink? A drink is technically 1 ounce of alcohol, which is equal to the following.

- 5 ounces red or white wine (100 calories)
- Flute of champagne (100 calories)
- 12 ounces malt liquor (1.5 ounces of alcohol; 175 calories)
- 12 ounces beer, regular or lite (110–150 calories)
- Shot of liquor (70 calories)
- Shot of liqueur (190 calories)
- Wine cooler (150 calories)

What about mixed drinks? Unless you are using water, club soda, or tomato juice as the mixers, the calories add up quickly, plus there is usually more than one shot or more than one type of alcohol in these drinks, e.g., martinis. You may be surprised to know that tonic water has the same number of calories as a cola drink even though it is not sweet. Some drinks may contain as many as 500 calories and don't make you feel full. In fact, alcohol can make you hungrier, so be careful. No drinking on an empty stomach! Watch what you mix with and how much alcohol you drink, and realize that if you do drink, you need to swap out calories from something else. Also, since alcohol is a diuretic, if you haven't had enough to drink during the day and then you ride, lose fluid, and then drink alcohol, you will be dehydrated.

YOUR DAILY FLUID DOSES

How much fluid do we need every day? The numbers listed below are *baseline* needs. Remember to figure in how much you need to hydrate your rides (see page 117 from Week 5).

> **For men:** 90–125 ounces per day, or 11–15 cups
>
> **For women:** 70 to 90 ounces per day, or 9–11 cups

If you eat more fruits and vegetables, you need less fluid because fruits and vegetables are about 85 percent water. So start munching! Try to space out your fluid intake evenly over the course of the day, including some at every meal and snack.

Here is a sample day for a woman who needs 11 cups of liquid a day. Each of the glasses is 8 ounces, or 1 cup.

- **WITHIN 1 HOUR OF WAKING:** water, juice, milk, coffee, or tea; at least one water
- **BREAKFAST:** water, juice, milk, coffee, or tea; at least one water
- **MIDMORNING:** water, coffee, or tea
- **LUNCH:** water, milk, coffee, tea, or soup
- **AFTERNOON:** water, tea
- **DINNER:** water, tea, or milk
- **EVENING:** water or herbal tea

If you distribute your fluid intake over the day, you won't need to drink copious amounts before bed and then spend the night traipsing to the bathroom.

Note: Track your fluid to see how much you are currently drinking during the day and make haste slowly. If you drink 4 cups a day now, don't drink 11 tomorrow! Gradually ramp up your fluids from 4 to 5 cups a day. Then, next week increase from 5 to 6 cups, and so on.

STRENGTHEN YOUR SUPPORT STRUCTURE

You need to take care of your bones and joints so you can get out there and ride. In Week 6, we discussed the importance of protein, not only for your muscles, but also for your bones and joints, so do make sure you include some protein as part of every meal or snack.

As a reminder, here are some high-quality sources of protein:

- Lean meat
- Poultry
- Fish
- Shellfish
- Eggs
- Soy foods
- Greek yogurt

- Low-fat milk
- Reduced-fat cheese
- Beans (such as chickpeas, black beans, kidney beans)
- Nuts and nut butters
- Seeds

How much protein? At least 0.5 grams per pound of body weight daily, but don't consume too much, which not only provides excess calories but also can be a bone robber. It is also needed to consume some fat as part of every meal. Fat and protein are important to transport vitamin D, which is a critical component of bone health. So don't adopt the "How low can I go?" strategy with fat intake. But do be selective. Choose fats such as olive oil, avocado, nuts or nut butters, or seeds, in small quantities. The omega-3 fatty acids in fatty fish such as salmon, sardines, herring, and halibut and in ground flaxseed are important for bone health as well as for reducing inflammation.

EAT YOUR IBUPROFEN?

We discussed this at length in Chapter 6, but it deserves another mention here. You may be tempted to pop ibuprofen or another nonsteroidal anti-inflammatory drug (NSAID) to ease the little aches and pains that can come with an active life—*don't*. These pills have become so ubiquitous in daily life that some people jokingly refer to ibuprofen as "vitamin I." Well, research is finding that NSAID abuse isn't a laughing matter. It not only can wreak havoc on your stomach, but also can actually hinder the muscle

FOODS FOR HEALTHY BONES

Put the following foods on your plate to build strong bones. Remember, the goal is not to add these foods on top of what you currently eat, but rather to swap them in so you keep your calories in check. For instance, dried plums can be a substitute for another fruit, or soy foods may replace chicken for your protein at dinner. Here's what to eat and why.

* Dairy foods contain calcium, vitamin D, and potassium.

* Dried plums contain boron, which is a mineral that increases the absorption of calcium.

* Fruits, vegetables, yogurt, beans, and nuts contain potassium, which increases bone mineral density and helps with calcium retention.

* Egg yolks contain vitamin D for bone and muscle health.

* Soy foods such as edamame, roasted soy nuts, soy milk, and tofu contain soy protein and also isoflavones to slow bone resorption.

* Beans, whole grains, leafy greens, nuts, and seeds contain magnesium, which helps with bone formation.

* Leafy greens, soy foods, and green tea contain vitamin K to produce osteocalcin and help with calcium absorption and bone mineral density.

* Citrus foods, citrus juices, tomatoes, and tomato juice contain vitamin D to help with collagen formation and the production of osteoblasts (bone cells).

recovery process. A far better choice is to seek out anti-inflammatory foods and drinks, as discussed on page 138. Many of these foods, such as fish and leafy greens, not only ease inflammation, but also help protect your joints and bones.

If you're not inclined to include a lot of those anti-inflammatory foods in your diet, you can supplement in some cases. You can take fish oil capsules for your omega-3s, if you don't eat fish. Krill capsules are available for those who are allergic to fish. Turmeric is sold in pill form as curcumin. Ginger is available in pill form as well. If you do decide to take supplements, make sure your health care provider knows what you are taking. Be aware, also, that both fish oil capsules and ginger are blood thinners. So if you already take aspirin, vitamin E, or warfarin (Coumadin), do not take any of the anti-inflammatory supplements before checking with your physician.

BYBO ASSIGNMENT FOR WEEK 8

For this week, I'd like you to do the following:

TRACK FLUIDS. Keep a tally of how many ounces you're drinking for the next day or so. Then calculate how much you need to add to reach optimum hydration (remember, if you're eating plenty of fruits and veggies, that counts) and make a plan for obtaining the proper amount. It may be as easy as keeping a refillable water bottle on your desk to sip from throughout the day.

Check your diet to make sure you're eating enough foods to support your bones and joints. If not, plan your substitutions using the recommendations above.

Consider increasing the amount of anti-inflammatory foods and fluids in your diet. If you can't seem to include at least a few a day, consider taking a supplement.

Secrets of Their Success

JAIME LIVINGOOD, 37

WEIGHT LOST:
6 pounds

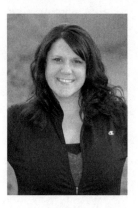

Jaime is surrounded by a community of cyclists. She volunteers at charity bike rides and local races. She is engaged to a cyclist. She loves cycling and follows cycling. She used to ride her bike everywhere as a kid, bought a bike as an adult, and has tried multiple times to be a cyclist herself. There's just been one thing holding her back: intimidation.

"I fell a lot when I was trying to get back into it and learning to clip in," she recalls. "It was also very intimidating to be around so many great cyclists. Guys and girls who 'just know' what they are doing. I knew that everyone had to start somewhere, but it felt like 'How will I ever get there? How will I ever get good enough to go on a ride with someone other than myself?' Everyone says, 'It's just like riding a bike. Oh, you never forget how to ride a bike.' Well, I used to ride my bike everywhere when I was 12—but I felt like I just had no idea what I was doing when I got back on my bike recently as an adult. Like, how should I be shifting, what should I be doing, how do I handle the bike? There's a huge difference between the bike you rode as a kid and the one you ride as an adult. And when I went out and got a road bike, it was way different from the hybrid bike I had before. I felt like I was out of control because it was so much lighter, faster, and so much more responsive. It was scary, especially out there alone."

In short, Jaime wanted "to feel more love for her bikes." She wanted to know how to ride and develop the confidence to ride with others. She also wanted to improve her fitness and drop a few pounds. She accomplished all the above.

"At first, getting on the trainer was what got me going again. But once I started riding outside more (with my faster friend Liz), all I wanted to do was ride outside. I didn't always remember the drills and intervals to the letter, but I did my best. One of the best parts, honestly, was sharing the ride with my riding partners Liz and Stacy. We practiced standing on inclines and shifting more, but it was also just so fun to talk and catch up and ride at the same time! I felt like we solved relationship problems, cleared our heads, and caught up on everything that we had missed in each other's lives—it was brilliant. There would be times I would forget my GPS and have no idea how long we were out or how far we went, because we were having so much fun.

"One funny thing that happened on a ride, I just have to share: I was out riding at the park the other evening, and I passed a dad and his son. Dad says to his son, 'See how fast that cyclist is going, you can go that fast.' I felt like a real cyclist, like I really knew what I was doing! Yay, me!!!"

Jaime, who has long suffered bouts of back pain, also really benefited from the supplemental core work. "My chronic back pain has all but gone away. I am able to get out of bed like a normal person, not like someone who needs to roll out of bed due to lower back pain. It's something I have dealt with pretty much my whole life, and it got worse when I tried running a lot. But with biking, my body feels so much better overall. It is like magic!"

Nutritionally, Jaime was pleased that the BYBO eating advice didn't force her to give up her one Diet Coke a day or make her eat foods that she didn't like. "Cooking and eating has never been my strong point, so having suggestions of what I can add to my fairly picky, limited diet was a blessing. One thing that helped for sure was the suggestion to get a blender and make some smoothies to get more fluids and fruits into my diet. I have been using frozen fruits, plain or vanilla Greek yogurt, fresh bananas, ice, and water."

She also started adding more protein to her snacks and meals, which helped immediately. "I don't feel like I am starving or depriving myself of anything really, and I'm still losing weight."

In the end, the pounds came off a bit slower than Jaime would have liked. But her history of thyroid problems has made weight loss a challenge, so she was grateful for the steady loss and is hopeful it will continue. "I know I still have a ways to go, but I weigh less than I did when I started. I feel stronger and more toned. My butt certainly feels more round and less flat, which I love because my flat butt has always annoyed me. My core feels stronger. And best of all, I'm ready and eager to keep riding and keep the gains coming!"

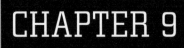

CHAPTER 9

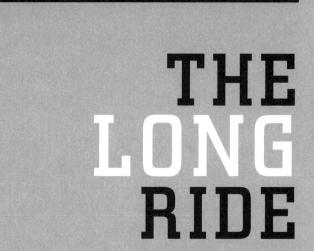

THE
LONG
RIDE

THERE'S NOTHING QUITE AS satisfying as what cyclists call the long ride. These can be destination rides—in my neck of the woods we do the Pagoda Ride, a 75-mile day that takes you out to a giant Japanese-style pagoda high up on a hilltop in the most unlikely place (Reading, Pennsylvania), and Hawk Mountain, a 90-mile bucolic round-trip that includes one of the longest climbs in our area. The ends of these journeys are nearly always the same. Everyone cracks a beer, digs into some food, and talks about how great it all was. You finish long rides with tired legs and a happy heart.

Of course, when you're just starting out, your long rides may not be anywhere close to 75 or 90 miles (heck, they may never be—and that's okay). They may be 20 or 30 miles. The long ride is relative and changes throughout your riding life. Our goal in this chapter is to equip you with the fitness and know-how you need to go as long as you want.

LAYER LIKE A WEDDING CAKE

Unless you ride long only on perfectly sunny summer days when there's no threat of "weather" in the sky, you'll need to learn how to layer. I've been on rides, especially in early spring, when the weather was capricious and unpredictable, where we rolled out under overcast 50°F skies and ended in 78°F sunshine. On the flip side, I've headed out in 70°F sunshine and ended up hauling arse out of the woods in 45°F degree pouring rain (I highly advise against that). In both cases, layering is essential.

Why is layering so important? Because layers trap your body heat between them, so you stay warmer during cool-weather rides. You can also remove a layer should the temperature rise unexpectedly. When done properly, your layers will also pull moisture away from your skin, as well as keep outside moisture from reaching your skin in damp conditions, to keep you dry and comfortable.

I often liken layering for a ride to a layered wedding cake—perfectly sweet when done right. Let's start with the foundation. A good base layer is a must. A high-tech fabric like a polypropylene-polyester blend will wick moisture away from your body. The problem is, many of these garments can trap odor and get pretty rank. You can go the natural route and choose a base layer crafted from merino wool. Unlike the itchy wool of the past, merino wool fabrics are soft on the skin, don't stink, and can keep your core warm on even the chilliest days. Whatever you do, *do not* wear cotton. It soaks up moisture without wicking, so you just have a heavy, cold shirt against your skin. Your base layer can be long- or short-sleeved depending on how chilly you expect it to be. Generally, once it hits the low 40s, I'm going with sleeves.

Next up is the midlayer. The role of a midlayer is to work with your base layer to wick away sweat and insulate your torso to provide warmth. For more mild conditions, a jersey and arm warmers will work just fine over a short-sleeved base layer. Again, when the mercury drops below 45°F (my personal threshold), I go with a long-sleeved jersey. An important point to watch for here is that your midlayer shouldn't be too tight. While cycling clothes are naturally snug, you need breathing room—literally—for layering to work because there needs to be some space to trap air and retain warmth.

Finally, top it all off with a little wind- and weatherproofing in the form of an outer shell. In milder weather, a vest is all you need. As it gets colder, a thin waterproof, wind-resistant jacket is the way to go. On cold-temperature starts, you can wear it out of the gate, then roll it up and stash it in your jersey pocket when the day warms up. Or, if you suspect you'll be out when the temperature starts to drop or you're going into the mountains where it might be very warm on a long climb and cold on the way back down, stash it in your pocket before you go just in case.

Pulling it all together: Layering for a 40°F ride might look something like the following:

- *Base layer.* A long- or short-sleeved undershirt (e.g., polypropylene-polyester blend or merino wool)

- *Midlayer.* A long- or short-sleeved cycling jersey, depending on the weight of your top layer.

- *Top layer.* A shell or jacket that's made from material that provides wind and water protection.

CRASH COURSES

They say there are two types of riders: those who have crashed and those who haven't . . . yet. I'm not sure I'd go that far. While most people I know have tipped over at least once (e.g., at a stop sign while learning how to use clipless pedals), I know plenty of riders who have not "crashed." So it's not an inevitability. But it is a possibility no matter how good a rider you are because random things can happen. I know a woman who was hit by a deer that had been hit by a car (she was fine; the deer not so much). So it's important to know what to do should you have an accident beyond a minor topple.

First and foremost, assess yourself. It's tempting to jump up and back in the saddle because you might actually feel fine. But don't let the adrenaline of the situation cloud your better judgment. Get off the road, take some deep breaths, and give yourself a thorough once-over. Scratches? Scrapes? Walk around. Anything really hurt as you move? Did you hit your head? If you hit it hard (check if your helmet is cracked), call for a ride and get yourself checked at the ER. Likewise, if you suspect anything is broken, call for help. You'd think you would know for sure if you've broken a bone, but trust me, that's not always the case. I hit a tree when I first started mountain biking, and four riders I was with stood around trying to determine if I had broken my collarbone. I had. But it was such a clean, stable break and I had so much adrenaline flowing through me, I could move easily, it didn't hurt that much, and I just couldn't tell.

Are you okay? Good. How's your bike? Start with the handlebars and work your way down the frame, drivetrain, and both wheels. Make sure the shifters and brakes are intact and functioning. Check your derailleurs (the rear is especially susceptible to bending or breaking). Spin the wheels. Do they wobble? Are any spokes broken? Examine the full frame for dings, dents, or cracks. If there's any damage, call for a ride. You don't want to risk crashing again because your bike isn't working properly. If you had a significant wreck, take the bike to your shop for a professional assessment or tune-up before taking it out again. Likewise, if you hit your helmet on the ground in the crash, replace it. It could be compromised even if it's not cracked.

If you find yourself riding a lot by yourself, I'd also recommend carrying a piece of identification with emergency information on it, just to be extra-safe. If you carry a cell phone, set up an ICE (in case of emergency) in your contact list—put your name, emergency contact's name, and their number in there. Or you can buy any number of Road ID products like bracelets and dog tag–style necklaces that provide your emergency info.

Of course, the best crash plan is one of avoidance. That's why there are so many Skill Drills in this book. Learning proper braking and cornering techniques goes a *long* way toward helping you keep your bike upright. If you're game, you can also do some bumping drills (I actually love these, but they aren't by any means essential). As you become more confident on your bike, go to a soft, grassy field with a friend, ride side by side at a comfortable pace, and practice gently nudging and bumping into each other. These drills build confidence and skill on several levels. For one, you learn how your bike behaves when it's acted on by an outside force. In one case it can be someone pushing you, but a strong crosswind can have a similar effect. You learn how to react (and not overreact) when something goes awry. Most important, you learn how to keep cool, keep pedaling, make minor adjustments with your steering, and stay upright and moving forward. You can read about how to do these things all day, but it's when you actually practice them that they become ingrained.

STRONGER LONGER

So we've spent the past several weeks working on cadence, bike handling, hills, speed, and of course fitness. Now it's time to start developing some muscular endurance. As the name implies, muscular endurance combines force and endurance, so you can turn a relatively hard gear at a high cadence for miles and miles. It's an often-overlooked component of cycling training, but it's one of the most essential for long-term cycling success, especially if your goal is to perform longer-distance cycling events like charity rides or even just weekend adventures with your friends. Obviously, you can't develop this in a week, but you can put the wheels in motion, so to speak, with tempo intervals like the ones you did in Week 5 and with the higher-gear, lower-cadence efforts you'll find on the following pages.

These efforts are a bit like strength training on your bike. They should feel hard on your muscles, but *not* on your knees. If you feel any twinges or discomfort in your joints, ease up on the resistance until you can pedal pain-free.

WORKOUT: BIG-GEAR CHURNING

// SKILL DRILL: Power Transfer

After weeks of working on speeding up your cadence, this week we'll be telling you to slow it down—just for short spells—as we help your legs tolerate putting out more force for longer periods of time. You can increase the force you put into your pedals without completely wearing out your legs by riding with your whole body. Practice on a slight incline. Shift into a fairly hard gear, tighten your abdominals, and, keeping your elbows close to your body, pull straight back on the bar with each pedal stroke. You should feel the power transfer from your arms through your core and into your legs.

BYBO CORE WORKOUT
(SEE PAGE 24 FOR EXERCISE DIRECTIONS)

Do the moves one after another like a circuit. Then repeat.

NOTE: New moves this week!

* Forearm Plank with Arm Raise
* Side Bridge Abduction
* Mountain Climbers
* Scorpion

BYBO STRETCHES
(SEE PAGE 36 FOR STRETCH DIRECTIONS)

* Figure 4
* Stork
* Windshield Wiper
* Cobra
* Prayer Pose

THE BYBO RIDE

TERRAIN: Flat to undulating

WHAT TO DO	INTENSITY	HOW LONG
Warmup	ZONE 1–2	10 min
Increase pace/intensity	ZONE 2	10 min
Find a slight to moderate incline and shift into a gear that is hard enough that your cadence slows to ~65–70 rpm. Assume the power position described on page 193 and pedal strong, seated.	ZONE 3–4	3 min
Coast back down; pedal easy	ZONE 1–2	2 min
Repeat power sequence 2 more times (or simply ride to another incline and repeat)		
Pedal briskly	ZONE 2	10 min

Finish with easy pedaling going home.

TOTAL TIME: ~50 minutes

Perform this workout 3 times this week.

TAKE HOME: These total-body workouts will improve your muscular endurance from head to toe. Again, it's important to pay attention to your weakest links while performing them, which are usually your knees. If you have any discomfort in your knees or other joints while performing muscular endurance efforts, shift into an easier gear until it goes away.

NOTE: *If you're already riding for longer than 50 minutes, simply extend the beginning or end of your ride or add another interval sequence.*

THE INSIDE RIDE

This week we'll give you a midride break to perform your four core moves. As in previous weeks, however, we'll mimic the outdoor ride and concentrate on muscular endurance, which will improve your ability to pedal strongly for a longer period of time.

WHAT TO DO	INTENSITY	HOW LONG
Warmup	ZONE 1–2	10 min
Increase pace/intensity	ZONE 2	10 min
Increase resistance enough that your cadence slows to ~65–70 rpm. Assume the power position described on page 193 and pedal strong, seated.	ZONE 3–4	3 min
Reduce the tension and pedal easy	ZONE 1–2	2 min
Dismount and perform the BYBO Core Workout		
Get back on the bike, spin for ~2 min, then repeat Step 3 muscular endurance sequence		
Pedal at a moderate resistance	ZONE 2	10 min
Pedal easy to cool down	ZONE 2 to 1	~3–5 min

Finish with some easy stretching after you're done.

TOTAL TIME: ~45 min

Perform this workout 3 times this week.

TAKE HOME: These total-body workouts will improve your muscular endurance from head to toe. As noted in the BYBO Ride section, however, if you have any discomfort in your knees or other joints while performing muscular endurance efforts, reduce the tension until it goes away.

WORKOUT LOG

Please log your workouts for the week.

WEEK 9				
BYBO Rides (including pleasure cruise) and Core Workouts	Date: Notes:	Date: Notes:	Date: Notes:	Date: Notes:
Cross-training and/or rest	Date: Activity: Duration:	Date: Activity: Duration:	Date: Activity: Duration:	Date: Activity: Duration:

ANY OBSTACLES? _____

ACCOMPLISHMENTS? _____

OTHER NOTES: _____

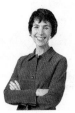

BIKE YOUR BUTT OFF! EATING PLAN: PUTTING THE BRAKES ON (EATING, THAT IS!)

So here is where Selene and I may seem to be at odds. She is having you do speed work as part of your training, but I want you to take it slow and easy when it comes to eating.

Why does it matter? Several studies have investigated "mindless eating" (when you eat without even being aware that you're popping food in your mouth, like at a party or standing at the kitchen counter with a bag of chips), the speed at which individuals eat, and what people are doing while they are eating, and they all have come to the same conclusion: Eating while multi-tasking, eating too quickly, and eating while distracted may take away from the satiety of the meal, and as a consequence, you overeat—without even realizing it. That's bad because you're eating too much, but also because when you eat too much without realizing it, you don't take measures to compensate for it by riding longer or eating less the next day, as you would when you knowingly overeat.

So let's work on your eating technique and surroundings. In Week 1, I asked you to log not only what you ate, but where you ate. Why? Because if you eat at the computer, while watching TV, while driving the car, or while on the phone, you are not and cannot be fully aware of what and how much you are putting in your mouth. That is why we are revisiting that strategy now. What has changed about your eating venues? Have you established different places and/or no-eating zones? What about the activities you are doing while eating? If it is anything other than chewing, you are going to be distracted. If eyes are engaged elsewhere, you lose the visual contribution to satiety associated with food.

What about your eating speed? Have you mastered the art of slowing down? Sitting down? Taking your time to chew and swallow? Take a look at Week 4, where I provided techniques for how to slow it down. Are you still practicing, or have you reverted to old habits? Be a hare on your bike if you like, but a tortoise at the table! This is especially important with indulgences. Think about holiday goodies: Halloween treats, Christmas cookies, Thanksgiving pies, and birthday cakes. It is really easy to wolf down these foods, which leaves you wanting more, eating more, and then storing more fat. Practice the art of the chew for a healthier, leaner, fitter you!

Now let's move ahead to the next skill I want you to address this week: hunger preparedness. Hopefully by now, you wouldn't ride without a helmet, or without rain gear when the weather is threatening, but do you always have some fuel and a water bottle with you on your rides? You should. Keep a stash of easily packable foods near your cycling gear. Good choices include nuts, dried fruits, honey sticks, or a medium-size energy bar (about 200 calories max). These foods are shelf stable and lightweight, so you can (and should) stash them in your pocket for each ride.

Why? Because you just never know. Case in point: You intended to ride for an hour, but it turns out to be a gorgeous day, you're feeling fine, and your riding buddy is up for more. But 2 hours in, you realize you don't have anything with you, and you are starting to get hungry and tired. The only thing you have is a water bottle, and so you end the ride before you wanted to because your legs are too fatigued. Don't let this happen. If you have fuel, you can refuel and ride on.

In addition to having food and fluid with you, prepare before you ride. We talked about fueling for rides in Week 5. But what about longer rides or races? Do you need to carb-load? *No*, because often that translates to carb-explode, as people feel compelled to consume a trough of pasta the night before a race. But endurance rides also mean you have to consume enough to help you ride long and finish strong, so what *should* you do?

I like the idea of fueling 3 days out from longer rides (like centuries), but remember that a little goes a long way. The purpose of fueling before an endurance ride is to stockpile carbohydrate in the liver and muscles so you have more energy available when you ride, and also to prevent your body from having to use its own muscle tissue as a fuel source during exercise.

How can you increase your carb stores without seeing the needle move up on the scale? You can't really in the short term, because if you eat a little more carbs, you will retain more water with those carbs, so the number will likely go up slightly. But it will drop back down again after your event. The trick is to not overload with carbs. I typically suggest that my athletes do the following, and again, this is *only* for very long rides (like centuries) or races.

On each of the 3 days before the event, add one additional carbohydrate food—and I am not talking scones, cupcakes, and candy bars. Try some of the following:

- 1 piece fruit (the size of a tennis ball)
- 1 serving cereal (look at the box!)
- ¼ cup dried fruit
- 1 slice bread
- ½ cup corn
- ½ cup pasta (measure after cooked)
- ⅓ cup rice (measure after cooked)
- 1 serving crackers (not a box!)

Add 8 ounces of fluid to every meal to which you add a carbohydrate-containing food. Resume your normal eating patterns after the ride is done.

For this week, I want you to continue to work on the speed and location of your eating. Be mindful of what you are putting in your mouth, see what is on your plate, and, honestly, you will find that you will be more satisfied for longer. Prepare your bag or pack with foods you can always have with you when you ride. Last but not least, as you prepare for the longer distances, remember to prefuel, and back it up a few days so you are not shoving food into your mouth the night before, or day of, your ride—or, worse yet, needing to end your ride because your legs have had it.

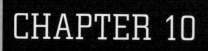

CHAPTER 10

GET OFF
YOUR BUTT

BY NOW I HOPE you're fully convinced of how good cycling is for your health. But I must tell you that if you want to lose weight and reap the full benefits of your riding, what you do during all those hours that you're not on your bike is at least as important as the time you spend on your wheels, especially if you have a desk job.

"Thanks" to modern technology, most of us are sitting, planted like potted ferns, for unprecedented amounts of time every day. With iPhones, iPads, laptops, notebooks, and electronic devices of every stripe, we can now work, play, shop, bank, pay bills, buy groceries, rent movies, and even socialize without ever so much as standing up. Well, here's a stat that might bring you to your feet. A survey of more than 6,300 men and women in the United States reported that we now spend nearly a full 8 hours a day—that's 56 hours a week—parked on our behinds.

That's bad. Really bad. New "inactivity research" (a growing body of science based on our increasingly sedentary lives) shows that when you sit for a few hours, your body literally starts to shut down, like a computer going to sleep, on the metabolic level. Fat-burning enzymes like lipoprotein lipase (LPL), which are responsible for breaking down triglycerides in your bloodstream, simply start switching off. Sit for a full day, and LPL activity drops to half its active healthy levels. The longer you sit without a break in the inaction, the deeper your body's sleep state becomes. Your circulation slows, your digestion becomes sluggish, and your calorie-burning metabolism dims to a flicker. Sit the majority of the day, and your scale will stay stubbornly stuck no matter how much you ride.

In fact, men and women who sit more than 7 hours a day are nearly 70 percent more likely to be overweight than those who spend fewer than 5 hours on their tushes, according to an Australian study. Prolonged sitting also raises your risk of diabetes, heart disease, cancer, and maybe even

Alzheimer's disease and depression. In a study of 168 men and women, Australian researchers reported that regardless of how much (or how little) moderate to vigorous exercise the volunteers did, those who took more breaks from sitting had slimmer waists, lower body mass indexes, and healthier blood fat and blood sugar levels than those who sat the most. A Canadian study of 17,000 men and women drew a starker conclusion: The longer you spend sitting, the more likely you are to die an early death no matter how fit you are.

As if that's not all bad enough, too much time on your seat also can hurt your cycling performance. When you sit for extended periods, your hip flexors and hamstrings become short and tight, while the muscles that support your spine become weak, stretched, and stiff, leaving you vulnerable to low-back pain on and off the bike.

TAKE A STAND

The first step to protecting yourself against the ill effects of too much sitting is standing up whenever possible. The mere act of getting up out of your chair is all it takes to break out of hibernation mode, switch on your fat-burning enzymes, boost your metabolism, and maintain healthy blood flow through your lower extremities. We're not talking about doing jumping jacks in your office; we're just talking about getting up.

Years back, I coauthored the book *Move a Little, Lose a Lot* with James Levine, MD, PhD, whose life's work revolves around studying the ill effects of sitting. He was adamant that simply standing up throughout the day could undo a lot of damage. "Simply standing burns three times as many calories as sitting," he told me over and over again. "And it's far better for you."

Whenever possible, walk. Get up once an hour and walk down the hall to talk to a co-worker you'd otherwise e-mail, go to the restroom, fill your water bottle—whatever you need to do, just get up and move. "It will help keep your hip flexors and hamstrings from becoming chronically shortened and tight," says competitive cyclist and chiropractor Ronald DeJong, another sitting expert I've worked with in McKinney, Texas. Plus, it's good for your spine. The best exercise for low-back health is walking because it places your discs under normal pressure.

Levine, who is so averse to sitting that he bolted a stand-up desk to a treadmill to create a "walking workstation," advocates three simple steps to keep you off your seat for prolonged stretches during the workday: Stand (and preferably pace) when talking on the phone. Walk to a colleague and talk face-to-face when a question will take more than one e-mail exchange to answer. Invest in a small notebook and do all your brainstorming on your feet. "By getting up and moving around more frequently, you'll also have

SITTING PRETTY

For many of us, long hours at a desk are a reality of life. Yes, we can stand up, maybe even walk, more often. But what is a desk jockey to do during all that mandatory chair time? Get some support for your spine.

Ideally, when you're sitting, you want to maintain the same natural S curvature in your back that you have when you're standing. That's the least stressful position for your spine. It's also hard to do without a little help, says Dr. Stuart McGill, of the Spine Biomechanics Laboratory at the University of Waterloo in Canada. "No matter how hard you try, it's the bottom two discs—L4 and L5—that are the ones that flex when you sit," he says. That's why he and other spine experts recommend getting a lumbar support pad to use when you're sitting.

McGill particularly likes the LumbAir, an inflatable lumbar pad that you can adjust to conform to the chair you're in and even the time of day. "Your spinal discs are swollen first thing in the morning, so you may find you need less padding early in the day than you do by later afternoon," he says. "You can pump it up as you need to throughout the day to maintain your back's natural curvature." Back experts also recommend putting a small footstool under your desk because elevating your feet helps to unload the spine.

more energy, so you'll be more likely to keep moving (rather than collapsing on the sofa) when the workday is done," he says.

While you're standing, do some stretching, particularly the extending variety. As a working cyclist, you likely spend a lot of time flexing forward over your handlebars as well as over your keyboard. Even on the busiest days, when you literally can't get away from your desk, stand up every half hour, put your hands on your hips, and bend backward looking at the sky. Then extend your arms overhead and take a deep breath to fully open your chest, engage your back muscles, and move your spine in a different direction to give your discs a break from being crunched in forward flexion.

USE THE FORCE

Ever notice how tired you get when you've been doing nothing but sitting around? That's the other problem with prolonged, uninterrupted sitting. It leads to more sitting because you're stuck in a pool of unmotivated, sluggish inertia. Well, here's where I encourage you to remember Newton's laws of motion that you may have learned in high school physics: A body at rest tends to stay at rest, and a body in motion tends to stay in motion unless the body is compelled to change its state.

That last part is really important. Motivation can plummet when you've been staring at spreadsheets all day. Sometimes the last thing you're going to want to do is change clothes, pump tires, and go for a ride. I fully understand. I love riding my bike more than nearly any activity I can think of, but sometimes I still have to force myself out of my comfortable office and out into the fresh air. But I'm never sorry I did.

Here's what I recommend for keeping your riding momentum rolling even when it's threatening to stall out.

CREATE A "DRIVE-THROUGH" SYSTEM. The easier it is for you to get out the door, the more likely you are to push through your inertia and get rolling down the road. Make it as simple as humanly possible by having all your cycling gear organized and ready to go. Even better, lay it all out—socks, jersey, sports bra or undershirt, shorts, shoes, bottles, and anything else you need—on a counter so you can slip out of your civvies and into your cycling kit in one smooth move.

MAKE THE 30-MINUTE PROMISE. So you may wake up and think, "I'm going to ride 2 hours after work today." Then 5:30 comes and you don't feel like you could ride 2 minutes, let alone 2 hours. That's when you need to do some bargaining with yourself. Tell yourself you'll do 30 minutes, a quick out and back just to knock out the cobwebs. I guarantee you that 15 minutes in, you won't want to turn around. And on the off chance you're so beat that you do, at least you got out and rode, which is always better than not riding at all.

MEET FRIENDS. It's clichéd advice at this point, but it works: Set a date to ride with a friend or two. That added layer of accountability gets you out the door even when you'd otherwise be sidelined by excuses.

WORKOUT:
MAINTAIN YOUR MOMENTUM

Okay, time to get back to the bike. This week we're going to work on making you a consistent cyclist. The most common mistake new riders (and runners and swimmers, etc.) make is starting out on a ride at full steam, only to fizzle out in an hour's time. Riding at a steady pace takes practice, which is what you're going to do with these cycling workouts.

ON THE BIKE

// **SKILL DRILL:** Steady as She Goes

Unlike in previous weeks, there won't be a lot of changing pace or cadence or doing intervals. Rather, I want you to warm up and then go right into a pace you feel you can sustain for the entire ride. While you're out there, practice the little skills like taking a drink and scanning for traffic, all while maintaining your pace.

BYBO CORE WORKOUT
(SEE PAGE 24 FOR EXERCISE DIRECTIONS)

Do the moves one after another like a circuit. Then repeat.

- Forearm Plank with Arm Raise
- Side Bridge Abduction
- Mountain Climbers
- Scorpion

THE BYBO RIDE

TERRAIN: Mixed terrain, including flats, undulations, and inclines

WHAT TO DO	INTENSITY	HOW LONG
Warmup	ZONE 1–2	10 min
Ramp up pace/intensity	ZONE 2–3	45 min

Stay in this zone, pushing into Zone 4 for short bursts if the spirit moves you, but keep your transitions smooth. Incorporate some of the stretching, shifting, and general riding skills you need for a long, mostly steady ride.

Finish with easy pedaling home.

TOTAL TIME: ~60 min*

Perform this workout 3 times this week.

TAKE HOME: These workouts are designed to be simple so you can practice maintaining a steady pace and effort while doing all the little things you need to do on your bike when you're on a longer outing.

NOTE: *If you're already riding for longer than an hour, go forth and pedal on!*

BYBO STRETCHES
(SEE PAGE 36 FOR STRETCH DIRECTIONS)

* Figure 4
* Stork
* Windshield Wiper

* Cobra
* Prayer Pose

THE INSIDE RIDE

This week we'll continue with the cardioresistance format, giving you a midride break to perform the four core moves. Once again we'll mimic the outdoor ride and concentrate on steady, extended efforts, which will improve your fitness for longer riding sessions.

WHAT TO DO	INTENSITY	HOW LONG
Warmup	ZONE 1–2	10 min
Increase pace/intensity	ZONE 2–3	15–20 min
Toss in bursts of speed and out-of-the-saddle efforts as you wish		
Reduce the tension and pedal easy	ZONE 1	1 min
Dismount and perform the BYBO Core Workout		
Get back on the bike, working back up to steady, moderate pedaling	ZONE 2–3	15–20 min
Pedal easy to cool down	ZONE 2–1	~3–5 min

Finish with some easy stretching after you're done.

TOTAL TIME: ~50–60 min

Perform this workout 3 times this week.

TAKE HOME: This workout stresses steady pedaling and building a solid fitness foundation.

WORKOUT LOG

Please log your workouts for the week.

WEEK 10				
BYBO Rides (including pleasure cruise) and Core Workouts	Date: Notes:	Date: Notes:	Date: Notes:	Date: Notes:
Cross-training and/or rest	Date: Activity: Duration:	Date: Activity: Duration:	Date: Activity: Duration:	Date: Activity: Duration:

ANY OBSTACLES? _____

ACCOMPLISHMENTS? _____

OTHER NOTES: _____

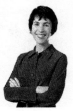

BIKE YOUR BUTT OFF! EATING PLAN: FOCUS ON FIBER, COLOR, AND REAL FOODS

Three weeks to go. So what are we going to focus on now? Fiber, plates full of color, and all the ways real foods make you a better, healthier cyclist for life. Oh, and because it's always somebody's birthday somewhere, I've included a little advice on eating on special occasions.

Let's start with fiber. It's filling and chewy and provides between-meal satiety. Even better, your body actually expends more calories to break down fiber into usable energy components than it does with a more refined type of carbohydrate. That means you burn more calories simply by eating fiber-filled foods than you do eating refined ones. That's one of the essential differences (there are a few) between eating a piece of fruit with skin and a bag of fruit snacks!

I am talking about *dietary fiber* here, though, not fiber pills, powders, or chews. You don't get the same benefit from washing down chicken nuggets with a glass of Metamucil. Where do you find dietary fiber?

Fruits	Nuts
Vegetables	Whole grains
Beans	Soy foods

Where don't you find it?

Meat	Sweets
Dairy	Oils and fats
Poultry	Beverages (unless you juiced whole fruits and vegetables)
Fish	

There are two types of fiber. Both are important for managing blood sugar, lowering cholesterol, and keeping your digestive system running smoothly.

INSOLUBLE: Helps with gut transit. You'll find it in the following foods:

- Skins of fruits and vegetables
- Bran in cereals and bread
- Nuts
- Seeds

SOLUBLE: Helps to manage blood glucose and lower blood cholesterol. It's found in the following foods:

- Flesh of fruits and vegetables
- Beans
- Barley
- Oats

HOW MUCH DO YOU NEED?

How much fiber you need depends on your gender and age. Men tend to be larger and need more. And we tend to need a little less as we age, when we typically need fewer calories and less food in general. The following chart is a good guide:

GENDER	< 50 YEARS	> 50 YEARS
Men	38 g/day	30 g/day
Women	25 g/day	21 g/day

What does that amount of fiber look like in a typical day of eating? It depends on the types of foods you pick. In general, high-fiber cereals like Bran Buds (13 grams per serving) are packed with it. Fruits and vegetables average about 2 to 3 grams per serving. Beans (kidney, black, baked) deliver about 7 grams per $\frac{1}{2}$-cup serving. Ideally you want to incorporate some high-fiber foods at every meal. Here are some ideas for meeting your fiber quota.

- Try a sprinkling of high-fiber cereal and berries on your morning oatmeal.
- Add some beans to a lunchtime salad.

- Try barley as an alternative to rice at dinner, and add some nuts and dried fruit for flavor and fiber.

- When you buy bread or cereal, don't just look for the words "whole grain" but also take a look at the nutrition facts panel and see how much fiber the product contains.

- To get the biggest bang for your fiber, choose fruits, vegetables, grains, and beans rather than fiber-enhanced yogurt, cookies, or beverages.

Make your plate pop with color. Colorful foods like fruits, veggies, and beans are chock-full of fiber and much, much more. The more different colors you can eat every day, the better. The pigments that give berries, peppers, leafy greens, carrots, and red beets their vibrant hues are some of the most potent antioxidants around. So aim to fill your plate with as much color as possible.

As a side (but very important) note, we hope that by this point everyone is hydrating enough because one of the roles of fiber is to pull liquid into the gut to soften the stool for easier elimination. This means that if you eat too much fiber and drink too little fluid, you can end up with trouble eliminating. So drink, drink, drink.

REAL FOOD VERSUS ENERGY FOOD

You've probably guessed by now that I am *all* about real food. The colors, flavors, and textures, not to mention nutritional value, cannot be replicated by processed foods no matter how hard the manufacturers try. And when you eat real food, you are more likely to be sitting at the table with utensils in hand and a plate or bowl in front of you.

So rather than engaging in drive-by eating out of a bag or a wrapper, do make an attempt to eat real food that you have cooked yourself. It honestly does not take that long to prepare, and if you are pressed for time, a salad from a grocery salad bar is much more satisfying and nutrient rich than an energy bar any day!

While we're at it, let's talk for a minute about "energy" products. Your body energizes with *food*. So even though there are several products that have the word "energy" plastered across the front, if they don't contain calories, they can't provide energy. Case in point—sugar-free Red Bull or 5-Hour Energy shots. Both clock in at under 5 calories, so no way can you be energized. Caffeinated, sure. But those are two different things.

I want you to think about what you snack on, what you pack when you ride, and work on making it more real. The following foods are good choices, and all are easy to pack as well.

- A Kind bar or Lärabar
- Whole grain crackers

- Trail mix
- Fruits (fresh or dried)

HOLIDAY AND SPECIAL OCCASION EATING

We think of the "holidays" as Thanksgiving and Christmas. But there are holidays (Easter, Passover, birthdays, etc.) year-round, so you need to always be prepared. I know, you're thinking that I am going to ruin your holidays, right? Wrong. My philosophy is that holidays are about enjoying the foods you don't get to have regularly, but with that being said, you don't have to eat the whole pie in one sitting.

So this is the time for swaps. If you want the pie, maybe you can compromise with a little less stuffing. Or perhaps have a smaller serving of mashed potatoes if you want dessert. And you can forgo the chips, pretzels, or dish of nuts that you could have anytime.

If you are celebrating a birthday, chances are that you are not going to put candles on a salad, so go ahead and have that piece of cake, but maybe you'll have the cake instead of something else, or plan your day so that you eat a little lighter at lunch and dinner to allow for the cake calories

It is all about skillpower, not willpower. You can talk yourself into enjoying within reason, or you can sabotage your good intentions by saying, "I have already eaten one cookie, so I might as well finish the plate."

Even if you overindulge on a holiday, it is not the end of the world, and the fact is that most people do eat more on Thanksgiving and Christmas. But it is what happens in the days leading up to and after the holidays that is more telling.

Are you overeating from Halloween to the end of the year? If so, can you get the Halloween candy out of the house so it stays out of your mouth?

If you are trying to be careful, do you really have to do the holiday baking? Maybe you can delegate or send people home with the leftovers so they are not there to tempt you? Also, you could always plan to take a longer ride. Not only do you burn more calories, but it gets you out of the house and away from the food

* * * * *

So for this week, here is your "to-do" list.

* Color up the plate.

* Add some fiber.

* Look at the labels and buy higher-fiber items.

* Include color at every meal—in the bowl, on the plate, or in the glass.

* Aim for more "real" food as a true source of energy.

* Start to strategize about the holidays and special occasions. What can you do to get you through?

Secrets of Their Success

JENNIFER ELDRIDGE, 41

WEIGHT LOST:
6½ pounds,
9.2 percent
body fat,
2 inches off her
waist

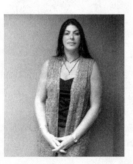

Jennifer didn't necessarily want to be a "cyclist" per se, but she liked biking. She owned an outside bike and a stationary bike and had access to a Spin bike through her gym. She felt, however, that she wasn't really getting what she wanted out of them. "I want to learn how to utilize all these bikes more effectively for maximum results," she told us.

We will tell you up front, Jennifer didn't lose all the weight she wanted, but she *did* steadily lose half a pound a week and came in for her final program follow-up positively glowing.

"I feel really great. My clothing definitely fits better, and I feel tighter all over. I definitely decreased inches in my overall body measurements, especially my legs and butt," she says. Part of what made her so successful this time around is being armed with the tools to make all the workouts she likes to do work better.

"I took your rules of engagement and used them for a variety of other workouts such as the elliptical trainer, stair stepper, treadmill, and my rebounder," she explains. "Toward the end I did about three BYBO routines a week, and 3 other days,

I alternated my workouts with the programs I mentioned, so I was doing something 6 days a week."

On the food side, Jennifer was already following a fairly strict regimen. "I don't take in any sugar. The only carbs I get are from sprouted bread, vegetables, and fruit. I eat no processed foods. I only eat meat, vegetables, fruit, seeds, nuts, and cheeses. The only indulgence I let myself have is on the weekend when I drink a little red wine."

Like many of us, however, Jennifer's distribution of her calories was skewed too heavily on the weekends, leaving her underfueled during the week. This can slow your metabolism and leave you relying on fumes for your workouts. "It's not unusual to see people eat pretty low calorically during the week and then much higher on the weekends, especially if they're drinking on the weekends," notes Leslie. "But if you're going to do that, you need to make adjustments."

Leslie advised trying to balance the calories by adding some sensible snacks during the week, particularly before workouts. She also recommended that Jennifer lower her fat intake on the weekends, especially if she wanted to indulge in some wine. "Alcohol is stored as fat in the body, so for weekend eating, if you are going to be drinking, keep other fat sources during the day lower to even out the calories from alcohol," Leslie advises. "For instance, instead of peanuts, perhaps have a bag of freeze-dried veggies to get the crunch you're craving, but with less fat and fewer calories. Or have an appetizer/snack of turkey pepperoni and pepperoncini instead of the cheese."

None of these were big, life-altering changes on either the exercise or the diet side. But that was the point. Jennifer just needed small adjustments that she could live with to get her on the road to slow and steady weight loss. Her transformation didn't happen overnight. But it happened and is still happening. And best of all, it's one she knows she can stick with for life.

CHAPTER 11

MILES AND MILESTONES

THE JOURNEY TO BECOMING a cyclist is just that—a journey. You start with that very first pedal stroke, filled with anticipation (and maybe a healthy dose of anxiety), and roll into a lot of unknowns. Along the way you have successes and setbacks. Depending on how much you know and how you come into the sport, you may hit a lot of setbacks, which is the reason for this book. As I mentioned in the introduction, so many people buy a bike with the best intentions of going somewhere new and exciting, but then cut their journeys short because no one ever showed them how to navigate the trip or what barriers they might encounter.

I also realized that cyclists generally travel along a very similar learning curve when they first start to ride, so if we could talk them through each step, we could make that curve less steep and more enjoyable. They'd be more likely to post some positive milestones and be encouraged to keep going. We were thrilled when that's exactly what our test panelists told us as they neared completion of the plan. One story that stood out as a shining example of how just a little guidance can completely alter the outcome of the journey was Sherrie Zacker's. Like so many aspiring cyclists, Sherrie started in a Spin class, got excited about cycling, bought a bike, and joined a group of friends for a ride, only to return feeling more deflated than a flat tire. She put away her bike and didn't ride again . . . until she found the Bike Your Butt Off! program. But we'll let her tell you in her own words.

In 2009 I started indoor cycling. I had no experience with any type of cycling other than when I was a kid. I started in the back row so no one would see me. I would watch the more experienced people in the front row and vow to be up there someday. Slowly I worked my way up to the middle, got cycling shoes that clipped in, then moved up to the front row. I worked on my form and speed and took on as many classes as I could. I wanted to ride outdoors with friends of mine, but I didn't have a decent bike and I heard so many things about accidents that it scared me. I was resigned to staying indoors.

I have a great group of friends who run and do triathlons. I am not a runner so I couldn't hang with them. But last spring they encouraged me to get a bike so I could ride with them when the weather was nice. One of them found a women's Cannondale [listed for sale] in a local cycling club's newsletter and I bought it. Before I could practice, my friends invited me for a ride. I went on a 30-mile ride out to Kutztown and back. At the first stop sign I clipped out with my right foot, but leaned to the left and fell over, knocking over two friends and getting a bloody chain bite on my leg. During the ride I spun too fast because I had no idea how to change gears. I tried to change gears going up a hill and knocked the chain off. I almost ran a friend over because I had trouble getting to the brakes. I swung wide on my turns and got in the way of others behind me. Basically, it was a disaster. I put the bike away and didn't ride it again.

When I heard about the BYBO project, I was so excited because I could learn how to ride correctly. The bike I bought had clipless pedals and that scared me to death. I was afraid of falling over again. I also didn't know how to navigate intersections and deal with traffic. The BYBO workouts taught me the fundamentals and forced me to get out, practice, and overcome my fears. Starting, stopping, scanning for traffic seem so basic, but it was a great way to start. I finally understand how to shift gears. THANK YOU! The concept of shifting prior to getting to the point where I needed was [the new gear] very helpful. I need more practice steering the bike with my body—I can't help but feel like I'm going to fall over—but I'll get there. I'm glad you encouraged me to take on the hills. I was avoiding them. I did have to get off and walk once or twice, but I got farther every time. Pushing the bike forward before returning to the seat was brilliant for me. Pushing down and pulling up while I pedaled was a much-needed reminder. I still need to work on my speed.

Thank you for being the inspiration I needed to get on the road with my bike. I now have confidence on my bike because I've learned the fundamentals. In fact, I've even taught my cycling friends a thing or two. Thank you for motivating and encouraging me. I can't wait for warm weather to get back outside.

RITES OF PASSAGE

As you can see, there are many rites of passage in becoming a cyclist: riding with people for the first time, clipping in to clipless pedals, doing that first big ride. But they don't stop after 12 weeks or 12 months or maybe even 12 years. The momentous occasions, both large and small, are endless once you hop aboard a bike and declare yourself a cyclist. Here are a few moments that the staff of *Bicycling* magazine, which you might imagine is filled with many seasoned cyclists, listed as some of the most memorable milestones in the cycling life.

- Realizing that the hill isn't in the way, it is the way.

- You go from one pair of shorts to a dedicated drawerful.

- Shaving your legs (for men; see "To Shave or Not to Shave?" on page 225).

- When "Thanks for the ride" goes from something you overhear to part of your lexicon.

- You see someone at the beach tanned low on the quads and biceps, and give him a nod of recognition.

- Bonking so bad you don't think you'll be able to make it home.

- Discovering how a convenience store cola can resurrect the dead.

When you hang out at the bike shop and no one expects you to buy anything.

When your bike computer registers triple digits for one ride.

Clearing a log on a trail.

Staying with the paceline long enough to take a turn at the front.

You're on the bike for the fifth straight day, and your butt doesn't hurt.

Your boss stops by to ask you to explain what's happening in the Tour de France.

You fix up your old bike to get someone into the sport.

Wearing out your first set of tires.

You ride through a pothole, and it's no big deal.

Getting hopelessly lost—deliberately.

Planning a riding vacation.

Seeing a sunrise from the saddle.

Wondering how the biggest local hill would rank on the Tour de France climb classification.

You got dropped, you flatted, bonked, got turned around—and when you got home you said you had a great ride.

Figuring out how to layer without overdressing.

Deciding which car to buy in part based on how it will carry your bikes.

Your first ride with a jersey instead of a T-shirt.

Riding on a day so cold the water in your bottle freezes.

Discovering that a shot of whiskey in each bottle keeps the water fluid.

Though you're not clear on exactly how to do it and unsure of the outcome, you manage to fix your first flat.

Naming a route.

Bumping elbows, then being relaxed enough to make a joke about it with the person next to you.

Developing that V of muscle definition on the back of your calf.

Espresso at the halfway point on a long ride.

Crashing and immediately asking, "How's my bike?"

Riding someplace you've always driven.

Outsprinting a crazed dog.

Feeling superstrong, then turning around for the ride back and realizing you had a tailwind.

Winning a town-sign sprint and remembering it forever.

You may not hit them all. But if you stay with the sport, I promise you'll hit a bunch and make many more of your own. In fact, our test panelist Jaime shared a few of hers with us that were simply too good to not pass along.

RIDING ON A HOLIDAY. "I realized that I had a 'first' on Thanksgiving morning when I got up early to ride with Liz. As ridiculous as that may sound, I have never gone out of my way to get up and do some sort of a workout on a holiday. I felt empowered! I felt great! And it made me feel so much better about potentially eating too much later that afternoon. I would have never done that before BYBO. Never."

NIGHT RIDING. "My first night ride [on trails] was amazing. I wasn't scared.

TO SHAVE OR NOT TO SHAVE?

Look closely at a pack of cyclists, and you'll see a few distinguishing characteristics that separate riders from runners and other active folks—hairless legs—on men. It's very common for male cyclists to shave their legs. Why? I think the most honest answer is that it's simply a long-standing tradition. But there are a few legitimate reasons to grab a Bic and shave those gams smooth. For one, it makes it easier to apply sunscreen and the warming oils (called embrocation) that cyclists sometimes wear to protect their legs when there's a chill in the air). It makes getting a massage—something you'll definitely want now and again when you start racking up the miles—more comfortable. It's easier to clean the dirt and gravel from road rash should you take a spill. And, well, to be completely honest, lots of guys just like to show off their newfound cycling muscle definition, which shaving does (bodybuilders do it for the same reason). You don't have to shave to be a cyclist, of course, but it is one way of showing that you're part of the club.

We just followed our lights and pedaled and talked and laughed. I never thought I would get that feeling, but I am beyond happy that I found it!"

GETTING BITTEN BY THE BUG. "I'm so comfortable on my bike now, I crave it. I feel like I have been bitten by the bike bug. I feel cranky if I haven't been on the bike after a few days. I am hoping the winter is quick and mild so that I can get out and ride more. Reading back through this makes me want to cry since I had such a great experience with the program. I never imagined that I could actually do it. I loved the journey that BYBO took me through both physically and mentally. Thank you!"

REAL-LIFE RIDING: INTERVAL MADNESS

So we've spent the past several weeks working on the skills and fitness you're going to need to succeed on your journey to become a cyclist—and on your cycling journey thereafter. But I will confess that this step-by-step approach, though effective, is a little artificial.

On any given ride, you'll likely encounter a chance to use most of the drills and skills you've practiced. Very likely you'll do a few of them one immediately after another. That inherent variety in conditions is what makes cycling such good all-around exercise. This week we'll do a little interval madness to sharpen your real-world fitness and skills and have a little fun.

WORKOUTS FOR // WEEK 11

WORKOUT: SPEEDPLAY!

> **// SKILL DRILL:** Rider's Choice!
>
> Work on your weakness. Still have a hard time making turns? Practice your counter-steering and tight turning in a parking lot. Take several minutes to hone those skills that still elude you.

THE BYBO RIDE

TERRAIN: Mixed terrain, including flats, undulations, and inclines

WHAT TO DO	INTENSITY	HOW LONG
Warmup	ZONE 1–2	10 min
Shift into a higher gear (but one that you can still spin at ~80 rpm) and ride tempo	ZONE 3	10 min
Shift into an easier gear; spin moderately	ZONE 1–2	2–5 min
Speedplay!*	ZONE 2–4	25–30 min
Ride easy	ZONE 1–2	5 min
Increase effort/pace	ZONE 3	3 min
Ramp up effort/pace	ZONE 4	2 min
Finish with one full-on effort	ZONE 4	1 min

Finish with easy pedaling going home.

TOTAL TIME: ~60–70 min**

Perform this workout 3 times this week.

*Perform intervals of various lengths and intensities. For example: Jump out of the saddle and sprint for 20 seconds in Zone 4, then coast and spin easy for 10 seconds; repeat this effort 8 times before changing the interval length and speed. Try to perform 4 different interval sequences.

**As always, feel free to ride for longer.

TAKE HOME: These workouts are designed to be hard, but they aren't supposed to be torture. So make sure you have some fun with them. If you have a like-minded workout buddy, bring him or her along!

THE INSIDE RIDE

This week we're going to break away from the cardioresistance format and keep you on the bike for the full workout before hitting the floor for your four core moves. As in previous weeks, however, we'll mimic the outdoor ride, which this week concentrated on speedplay—a fun, spirited mix of intervals meant to condition you for whatever the road or trail throws your way.

WHAT TO DO	INTENSITY	HOW LONG
Warmup	ZONE 1–2	5–10 min
Increase the resistance (but one that you can still spin at ~80 rpm) and ride tempo	ZONE 3	5–10 min
Shift into an easier gear; spin moderately	ZONE 1–2	2 min
Speedplay!	ZONE 2–4	20 min
Perform intervals of various lengths and intensities. For example: Increase resistance and jump out of the saddle and sprint for 20 seconds in Zone 4; lower tension and spin easy for 10 sec (repeat 8 times).		
Spin moderately/briskly	ZONE 1–2	5 min
Increase resistance/effort	ZONE 3	3 min
Ramp up effort/pace	ZONE 4	2 min
Finish with one full-on effort	ZONE 4	1 min
Pedal easy	ZONE 2–1	5 min

Total time: ~60–70 min

Perform this workout 3 times this week.

Take home: These workouts are designed to be hard but fun—make sure you have some fun with them. Music helps!

WORKOUT LOG

Please log your workouts for the week.

⟳	WEEK 11			
BYBO Rides (including pleasure cruise) and Core Workouts	Date: Notes:	Date: Notes:	Date: Notes:	Date: Notes:
Cross-training and/or rest	Date: Activity: Duration:	Date: Activity: Duration:	Date: Activity: Duration:	Date: Activity: Duration:

ANY OBSTACLES? _____

ACCOMPLISHMENTS? _____

OTHER NOTES: _____

BYBO CORE WORKOUT

(SEE PAGE 24 FOR EXERCISE DIRECTIONS)

Do the moves one after another like a circuit. Then repeat.

- Forearm Plank
  with Arm Raise
- Side Bridge Abduction

- Mountain Climbers
- Scorpion

BYBO STRETCHES

(SEE PAGE 36 FOR STRETCH DIRECTIONS)

- Figure 4
- Stork
- Windshield Wiper

- Cobra
- Prayer Pose

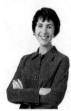

LESLIE'S LESSONS

BIKE YOUR BUTT OFF! EATING PLAN: CRAVINGS, SNACKING, OVEREATING—OH MY!

Wow, Week 11 already. Time flies when you are on the bike, as well as at the table! This week Selene mentioned that becoming a cyclist is a journey—one that is ultimately rewarding but not always smooth sailing. So it is with the journey to become a healthy eater. There will be potholes and pitfalls, sometimes daily. But the more skills you have to negotiate them, the less of an obstacle to progress they'll be. This week's goal will be providing you with the skill set you need to deal with some of the most common bumps in the healthy-eating road—cravings, snacking, and overeating after exercising.

QUELL YOUR CRAVINGS

If you think you crave chocolate because you have a magnesium deficiency, think again. Nice try, but wrong answer. Cravings are *normal,* and a combination of brain want and body desire. This one-two punch makes cravings feel nearly insurmountable at times. But people do try . . . and try again to defeat them. Many clients I see try to employ these strategies to deal with cravings.

1. Eat around it.

2. Ignore it.

3. Give in and go overboard with food intake.

Here's why none of them ever work—and what does!

SCENARIO 1

You really want some chips, but you say to yourself, "Too fattening, I will have an apple instead." *Hello*—apples are sweet and crunchy—not savory, salty, and crispy. Of course the apple doesn't do it, so you eat rice cakes, then some nuts, then a few carrots, and maybe even some crackers, and *you still want the chips*!

So rather than eat around them, have some, but in the stated serving size (yes, count out 10 or 15 chips or whatever the bag indicates), in a bowl, sitting down and enjoying them. Trust me, you will consume far fewer calories *and* be more satisfied.

SCENARIO 2

You are on your way to lunch and spy a birthday cake in the office pantry. It looks good. Everyone is eating it. You are hungry. You are vulnerable. It is nearly impossible not to think about, let alone eat, the cake. What to do? *Get lunch.* You can't expect yourself to ignore cravings when you are genuinely hungry. So go and eat a proper lunch. When you come by the pantry again, ask yourself if you're really hungry or if you can pass it up. Give yourself

10 minutes, and if you still want the cake, have a small slice. Chances are good that by the time 10 minutes go by, you'll be wrapped up in something else and make it through the rest of the day cake-free.

The dreaded "I have already blown it, therefore, I might as well eat the whole [bag, box, carton, container]." This is the door you don't want to pick. Okay, everyone has days when they are not perfect with eating, and sometimes those goodies are calling your name. But if you consistently think of having one treat or indulgence as blowing the whole day, you will blow most days. So what can you do? *Swaps!* If you eat the cookies, then how about lightening up on the next meal, cutting back on the pasta, rice, or potatoes while emphasizing the lean protein and veggies? Healthy eating is not an all-or-nothing journey. It can't be. Even one day of gluttony does not ruin your health. So get all those negative and sabotaging thoughts out of your head. Those attitudes are what make you overeat, not that single cookie at lunch.

SNACK SMART

Snacking has become something of a great American pastime. It is something we all like to do. But when you think snacks, what comes to mind? A pork chop, a salad, and a baked potato? I didn't think so. More like chips, cookies, candy, popcorn, pretzels—basically, treats. Oftentimes, it is not the meals that are the issue when you are trying to lose weight, but what happens in between. Even when snacks are small in size, they can end up on your thighs if you aren't careful.

I recommend eating three full meals a day, so you're not as tempted to snack in between. Then have these strategies in place to play it smart when you do want to snack.

1. Limit the snackable items you keep around. The more choices you have available, the more will end up in your mouth.

2. Don't be misled by 100-calorie snack items; they are pricey and unsatisfying because they tend to be highly processed, empty-calorie types of foods. Instead, make your own, such as the following:

   - Celery and 1½ tablespoons peanut butter
   - 2 Laughing Cow cheese wedges and an apple
   - 100-calorie bag of popcorn (the one exception to the avoid-100-calorie-snack-items rule!)
   - Smoothie of 4 ounces skim milk, ½ cup frozen berries, and 2 tablespoons Greek yogurt

3. Portion out your snacks ahead of time. Buy small reusable containers for your snacks.

4. Try to incorporate fruits and/or veggies into your snacks whenever possible.

5. If you are truly hungry, make your snacks more like mini meals: a cup of soup, half a sandwich, or a bowl of cereal.

6. Sit down and eat your snack so you know you have eaten.

7. Make sure you count the snacks in your daily food tally.

8. Snack only when you need it most. If it's very close to your next meal, wait.

9. Go for something different. If you always choose sweet snacks, try savory; if you are a crunchy, salty person, try smooth and creamy to change it up and perhaps be satisfied with less.

10. Lighten up on the beverages to save some calories. Instead of sweet teas, juices, and/or sodas, go with herbal tea (hot or iced), vegetable or tomato juice, or sparkling water with lemon, lime, or orange slices.

Again, don't forget to list your snacks in your food logs. Sherrie, who made such brilliant progress in her cycling journey by learning how to negotiate all those common obstacles, found that she could make equally good progress in her healthy-eating journey by doing the same. Her words:

I thought I had a pretty good diet, but I learned so much during this process, especially how much I was actually eating—everywhere! I learned to eat slower and most importantly incorporated "No Eating Zones," like at work and in front of the computer. I concentrated on sitting and enjoying my food in a relaxing way. I learned to eat full meals so I don't get hungry and snack or graze. I came to realize that I had such a hard time keeping my food diaries because I was eating on a constant basis. No more.

AVOID OVEREATING AFTER EXERCISING

In Week 6 we talked about recovery eating and why it is important to replenish after a hard ride, but a little goes a long way. So many times my athletes and clients tell me they are frustrated that they are not losing weight even though they exercise regularly. Then I ask them to log every morsel they eat, and I see they are effectively wiping out their workouts by eating too much food afterward.

Time for a reality check. Although you do burn calories when you ride, it is really easy to put those calories back and then some if you aren't careful. This is why I always use the phrase "Less is more." You can prevent overeating after riding by properly fueling during your rides. This means taking in small amounts of carbohydrates in every hour you ride after the first hour. Thirty grams is what I am talking about! That is *not* a lot. You get that much carbohydrate from any one of the following:

16 ounces sports drink

1 package Gatorade chews

3 honey sticks

1 gel pack

If you take in more than that, you may not lose weight, and may actually gain.

* * * * * *

When you are done riding (again, this is only after long or hard rides), you don't require a lot of food to start the recovery process. As I mentioned in Week 6, you need no more than the 200 calories in, for instance, any one of the following:

* A small bar (Luna, Lärabar, Kind bar)

* 10 ounces low-fat chocolate milk

* 1 cup cereal with $\frac{1}{2}$ cup skim milk

* Half a turkey sandwich

* 100-calorie yogurt with fresh fruit added

* $\frac{1}{3}$ cup mixed nuts and dried fruits

CARBS: THE GOOD, BAD, AND UGLY

While we're talking about fueling, refueling, and the potential for overeating, we need to address carbs because they're the easiest of the foods to overeat. There are many choices when it comes to carbohydrates. Choosing wisely will go a long way in preventing overconsumption and weight gain.

BEST CHOICES

- Fruits
- Vegetables
- Milk or yogurt
- Whole grain bread
- Corn or whole wheat tortillas
- Brown rice
- Pasta (whole wheat or a small portion of white)
- Cereal
- Plain popcorn

Focus primarily on the ones that have fewer calories and more nutritional value.

- Fruits and vegetables provide carbs, fiber, fluid, vitamins, minerals, and phyto (plant) nutrients.
- Milk and yogurt provide carbs, protein, vitamins, and minerals.
- Whole grains such as brown rice, oats, corn (including popcorn), barley, and whole wheat bread provide carbs, protein, vitamins, and minerals, and phyto (plant) nutrients—but you still have to watch how much you eat because they're easy to overdo.

NOT SO HOT

- Crackers
- Pretzels
- Buttered popcorn
- Sweetened beverages
- Syrups, sugar, honey (in large amounts)
- Desserts
- Candy
- Alcohol

I am not saying you should never have these items, but unlike other carb choices, what do we get from these? Not much that's good for you.

- Crackers, pretzels, and tortilla chips contain mostly carbs, fats, and salt.

- Sweetened beverages are nearly pure sugar.

- Syrups, sugar, honey—again, pure sugar.

- Desserts and candies are carbs plus fat.

- Alcohol is a carb, yes, but it's stored in the body as fat.

If you think your diet is still a little carb heavy, here are some creative ways to trim down slightly while still getting the fuel you need to ride.

- If you eat granola, how about having one-third granola and two-thirds flake cereal?

- If you eat a large serving of pasta, how about having less pasta and adding some vegetables and lots of sauce?

- If crackers and hummus are your thing, how about switching half the crackers for veggies for dipping?

Pulling it all together, this is what I would like you to do this week.

1. Work on your craving strategies. How will you manage them?

2. Write out a smart snacking list *and* the proper portion sizes.

3. Determine if you are eating too much on the bike or when you're done, and take a little off the top.

4. Think about your carbs: Be a smart carb chooser to be a better weight loser.

CHAPTER 12

DON'T STOP NOW!
HIGHLY EFFECTIVE HABITS OF LIFELONG CYCLISTS

WELL, HERE WE ARE, the end of the road on the BYBO plan. But hopefully, like Jaime, Sherrie, James, and our other panelists, it's just the beginning of the road for you as a lifelong cyclist. You have the foundation you need to grow. All you need to do is build a little bit at a time—ride more when you can, continue structured training, maybe invest in some cool new gear, and find new ways to keep the weight coming off as you continue along your journey in the sport.

To help, this chapter is chock-full of advice that every seasoned cyclist should know—and many have had to learn the hard way. Think of it as receiving the kind of golden nuggets about everything cycling—training, technique, lifestyle tips, you name it—you'd get from professional cyclists, coaches, exercise scientists, and all the best members of your local cycling club, all in one place. Take it. Share it with your friends. And, above all, use it and ride lots.

THE 10 COMMANDMENTS OF TRAINING

It seems appropriate to start this chapter with a little piece I compiled for *Bicycling* magazine years back on the best training advice I had ever heard, dished out, and tried. When you get to the point where you want to take your cycling to the next level—going faster and/or farther—you need to train (which, of course, is exactly what you've been doing these past 12 weeks). As you go forth in your training, remember these rules.

1. **HAVE A PLAN.** Winging it is fine sometimes, but it doesn't quite cut it when you want to achieve something great. Truly remarkable accomplishments, whether finishing your first century (100-mile) ride or lining up for your first race (yes, it could happen), require careful planning and execution.

2. **BE PREPARED TO SCRAP THE PLAN.** You're scheduled for 3 sets of high-speed spin-ups, and your legs feel like they're churning through wet cement. Try a couple efforts to see if they come around. If they do not, your body is telling you it hasn't recovered from your latest effort. Take the day easy and hit it hard tomorrow instead. Your plan should be etched in clay for molding it to your needs, not in stone for hammering yourself with.

3. **RIDE AT THE EXTREMES.** Many cyclists never go hard enough or easy enough to make big gains. Instead, they spend most of their rides going comfortably hard. Once a week, go so hard your eyes hurt. Follow it with a ride so slow the snails yawn. The combination makes legs strong.

4. **BE TRUE TO THYSELF.** Most cyclists are pack animals by nature. Enjoy the camaraderie, but don't let your training goals get trashed by the constant KOM (king of the mountain) contests, town-sign sprints, and all-hard, all-the-time mentality of the group. If you can't trust yourself to sit in and go easy when you need to, go alone.

5. **DO WHAT SUCKS.** You hate climbing because it's hard for you. You should climb because it's hard for you.

6. **THINK PROGRESSIVELY.** Do more than log miles. Don't leave behind the drills from the past 12 weeks just because the plan is over. Do intervals, cadence rides, and other specific workouts designed to progressively challenge your body in different ways from week to week. Give every ride a goal.

7. **MAINTAIN THE HUMAN MACHINE.** Keep strengthening your core and other stabilizing muscles. Keep stretching. By keeping your supporting muscles strong and joints flexible, you can avoid an achy back, tight hip flexors, and other overuse injuries that can weaken even the strongest cyclist.

8. **TRAIN YOUR BRAIN.** Your body can do more than you think. Convince it using your brain, through positive self-talk and visualization. You'll be surprised by what you accomplish when you say you can.

9. **EAT.** Fuel is everything for accomplishing big goals like 100-mile rides or multiday charity rides. Train your belly like you do your legs. Fuel your workouts with the same foods you eat on event day. You'll ride faster in practice and digest better when it counts. Don't be afraid to experiment. There are dozens of different energy concoctions for a reason. No one thing works for everyone.

10. **ENJOY THE RIDE.** You have a job. Presumably, riding's not it. Work hard at it. But never make it work.

ADD THESE TO YOUR TRAINING LOGS

Recreational cyclists often think they can't get overtrained or "get stale," as it's often called, because they don't ride enough. Heck, they don't even know what being overtrained means. Fact is, recreational cyclists can be at special risk for overtraining— having persistently heavy legs and feeling constantly tired— because they're often trying to squeeze their cycling training into hectic lives crammed with other obligations.

THE BEST WAY TO STAY FRESH: Pay attention to your moods, says John Raglin, PhD, professor of kinesiology at Indiana University, Bloomington, who recommends "mood monitoring" to detect creeping staleness before it becomes a full-blown problem. Staleness is the end result of a string of biological disruptions like rising stress hormones, dips in feel-good neurochemicals like serotonin, and muscle breakdown. Your moods are like canaries in a coal mine, giving you an early indication of when these biological factors are heading south. "With hard training, you're bound to feel tired and maybe a little low," says Raglin. "But your mood should improve with rest and you should be ready to go by the next session. If your mood is persistently low, you need to pull back until you feel better. Overtraining is always a function of too little rest and too much training."

MAINTAINING BALANCE

Cycling is about balance, both on and off the bike. And when you have a job and kids, it can be tricky to keep it all upright and rolling in the right direction. For myself, it's a balancing act between my own riding, training, and racing and my husband's riding, training, and racing. We have a 10-year-old daughter who prefers other activities to cycling, so we need to be sensitive to what she wants to do and be sure to spend time with her as well.

For us, it just means a little advance planning. On weekends we often take turns, one of us riding first thing in the morning, one when the other comes back, then doing family stuff for the rest of the day. Other times we'll hire a sitter for a couple of hours so we can ride together, or we'll go when our daughter is at a friend's house or with her grandparents. Knowing that hundreds of professional riders face the same issues, I asked a few coaches and professional and recreational racers how they keep it all in balance. Here's what they said.

TURN DOWN THE VOLUME. "During times of high family obligations, forgo the long rides and focus on getting out a little bit every day for drills and intervals," says Andy Coggan, PhD, USA Cycling scientific advisor and national-caliber masters racer. "Physiological adaptations to training only occur in response to an overload, so if you are going to make any forward progress with limited time invested, you need to be certain that you are appropriately stressing your systems." In other words, when time is short, go hard more often.

LET GO OF THE SMALL STUFF. I swear by this. So does my teammate Cheryl Sornson, mountain bike racer for Team CF, National Ultra-Endurance Women's Open champion 2008 and 2012. "Think of time in chunks and schedule in the big stuff and then let the little stuff find its way in. Be realistic about demands on your time and look long-term, not just day by day or week by week. Maybe during the season the house is a bit unkempt, but during off-season you take some time to prepare the house for the next season. Decide what is really important and cut out little things that waste your energy and time."

HIT THE HIGH NOTES. The big thing is being flexible with your schedule, says David Wiens, mountain bike legend and six-time Leadville 100 winner. "Once you have kids there are so many variables you can't control. They get sick. They have snow days. They can toss all kinds of wrenches in your schedule. Try not to get too tied into getting in a particular ride on a particular day. Rather than being set in stone on a weekly schedule, aim to hit all the high notes—your long ride, your intervals, and so on—and you should be good to go. Being mentally flexible will also help you in whatever events you do."

PUT 'EM IN TOW. "I'm a big believer in taking the kids along," says Marla Streb, Luna Women's Mountain Bike Team member and former single-speed world champion. "When my kids were young, I did most of my riding with them in the Chariot trailer."

SUPPORT YOURSELF AND RECRUIT SUPPORT. "You can make a lot of excuses for not riding once you have kids—too tired, too busy, not enough time, and so on," says Danelle Kabush, two-time Xterra world champion with Luna Xterra. "But I believe I'm a better mom and wife in the end because training allows me to take a little time to myself each day, stay healthy, and be a role model to my daughter," she says. It takes commitment and making it a priority while respecting the demands of family life. You can't do it alone! Reach out for the support of others—your spouse, parents, in-laws, and babysitters. With motivation, commitment, support, and creativity, you can train without sacrificing all your family time.

GET THEM INVOLVED. Lots of charity events have shorter family-friendly distance options, and even races have kids' heats, where young riders can get a taste for how much fun it can be to pedal with a purpose. So if they're game, make them part of the team. They'll have fun, you'll have fun, and even better, you'll be sharing something you love.

GO BY BIKE!

Our test panelist Becky rides nearly 20 miles a day many weeks without ever "going for a ride." How's that? She commutes to her job in Pittsburgh by bike.

"It's 8 to 10 miles depending on how I go in," she says. "I take the bike lane in the morning because it's a nicer ride. Then I'll take the short way home, which means a shorter but harder ride because there's an intense hill at the end of it."

Commuters like Becky enjoy the fact that instead of sitting inside a metal box, agitated by traffic, barely noticing your surroundings, riding allows you to soak in the blooming flowers in springtime, feel the morning air and sunshine, and arrive at work with a smile plastered on your face and your brain pumped with endorphins and ideas. And, as she discovered, you can lose weight just by going back and forth to work every day.

Jerry Edelbrock, a 50-something cyclist living in San Francisco, described the beauty of bike commuting perfectly: "I look forward to going to work as much as coming home, and I feel good about whatever I have to face." Though he's been making the 16-mile trip to and from San Francisco's financial district for more than a decade, it still makes him giddy to pedal over the Golden Gate Bridge, especially during full moons in the wintertime. "The moonlight over the water is emblazoned in my memory. It's unbelievable."

Now a confession: As much as I ride my bike—and I ride it an awful lot—I don't use it for transportation as often as I should, which is something I've been trying to be better about over the years. I work from a home office, so a daily commute isn't in the cards. But I also live in a town and am no more than 1 to 3 miles away from the grocery store, the bike shop, and the *Bicycling* magazine offices. I've discovered that depending on where I need to go, it's often faster by bike. And statistics show that even longer-distance trips really don't take that much longer because you spend less time at a standstill.

As mentioned earlier, trips of less than 3 miles are often faster by bike, and those 5 to 7 miles in length take about the same time by bike as by car. Longer trips will take more time than in a car, of course. But even if you spend an extra 20 minutes or half hour riding, it's always more pleasant than sitting in a car.

And, hey, it's better for you and the environment. Census figures show that we Americans spend an average of almost an hour a day on our daily commutes. Tack on to that the 38 hours a year we spend stuck in snarled traffic (a figure highway experts warn could quadruple in coming decades), then figure in our daily errand-driving miles (which have more than doubled since 1969), and we practically live in our bucket seats. If you spend even some of that daily drive time pedaling instead, you'll reap numerous rewards, including the following.

BETTER BODY. Ride your bike to work like Becky, and you no longer need to make time to exercise. Rack up just 3 hours of riding time per week, and you can slash your risk of heart disease and stroke in half. Plus, you'll lose the gut and unwanted flab—no diet required.

MORE MONEY. The average annual cost of keeping an automobile running: at least $3,000. The cost of running a bike for a year: less than $300. The joy of saving more than two grand this year: priceless.

CLEANER AIR. The number of communities that will fall out of compliance with the Clean Air Act is expected to triple within a decade. Motorized vehicles are responsible for 70 percent of the carbon monoxide, 45 percent of the nitrogen dioxide, and 34 percent of the hydrocarbons people produce. Riding a bike is a simple way to improve the environment.

It's also the perfect time to start commuting, as many communities around the United States are striving to make themselves more bicycle friendly by installing miles of bike lanes, wider shoulders, and bike racks for parking. If you're a new commuter, you'll likely have a few logistical details, such as routes and carrying bags, to sort out before actually making the trip. Here are some tips for making your maiden voyage smooth sailing.

SELECT YOUR ROUTE

Depending on where you live, you may follow the roads you drive on your bike, or you may need to find a route that avoids highways or unsafe roads. Your local bike shop can assist you in choosing the best routes to your destination. It also may have bike maps that show bike-friendly routes in your region, so you can try several different routes.

PROTECT YOUR SKIN

Pedaling away the hours in the great outdoors is wonderful for your body and soul, but it can be a little tough on the skin. Sun, wind, and chafing all can take their toll. Here's how to keep yours protected.

WEAR SUNSCREEN. A funny thing about riding is that you often don't feel like you're getting burned until it's too late, likely because of the cooling breeze you create as you slice through the air. Well, you can't ride away from the sun's dangerous UV rays, so protect yourself with a sweatproof, waterproof, long-lasting sunscreen. I like the spray-on kind so I can cover every inch of exposed skin even when there's no one around to get my back.

CONSIDER SOME SKINS. If you're particularly sensitive to the sun, consider a pair of summer sun sleeves, like those made by Pearl Izumi. They have UV protection built into the fabric and are designed to keep you cool in the hot summer sun.

BUTTER 'EM UP. Some people can ride their whole lives without ever chafing or succumbing to saddle sores. Others simply have more sensitive skin. If you're in the latter camp, buy a little chamois cream like Chamois Butt'r and rub it on your nether regions and upper thighs before you ride. It'll prevent chafing and saddle sores on long rides. Even if you never have to use it, have some on hand for days you might be caught in the rain. Wet chamois equals a sore, chafed butt. I don't typically need chamois cream, but I always wear it if there's a chance of rain.

LOSE THE SHORTS. There are riders who will sit around in their clammy chamois for hours after the ride is over. Kindly don't be one. Once you're off your bike, lose the shorts as soon as you can, wipe down with some baby wipes (or at least a little water), and pull on some clean clothes. Your behind will thank you.

COVER UP WHEN IT'S COLD. Cold, dry air can not only leave your skin dry and cracked, but also be hard on your joints and connective tissues—especially your knees. The cartilage in your knees is elastic when warm but a little brittle when cold. Keep your hinges toasty and fluid with leg warmers or petroleum jelly when the temp dips below 70.

Another option is to explore any one of the online mapping services like Google Maps and MapQuest, which allow you to investigate all the back roads between you and your destination.

"RIDE" WITHOUT A BIKE

Unless you're paid to ride, there are going to be times when life forces you to spend more time away from your bike than you'd like, whether it's a family vacation to Disney World or a prolonged business trip. Personally, I think cross-training is a good idea anyway, but when you can't ride, it's essential for maintaining your fitness. Just what type of cross-training is best is a matter of debate.

One school of thought says that your cross-training activity of choice should be entirely different from cycling—an activity like running or swimming that uses completely different muscle groups and theoretically should help keep you more balanced in the long run. The other school believes that whatever noncycling activities you do should be as close to cycling as possible to provide more sport-specific fitness. Personally, I ride the fence between the two.

Generally speaking, while I think that cross-training ought to provide balanced fitness and strength, I also believe that it's best when it complements cycling at least indirectly. Here are some cross-training activities that do just that.

HILL RUNNING. Watch your legs as you're running uphill, and you'll see they look an awful lot like your legs when you're riding a bike. Likewise, when you're out of the saddle climbing uphill on your bike, your legs will look a lot like you're running uphill. If you don't have a lot of time, doing a short, hilly run or hill repeats (where you simply run up the same hill) is a great way to boost your strength and fitness fast. The problem with running uphill (as opposed to riding uphill) is you then have to get back down the hill, and running downhill can be hard on your muscles and joints if you're not used to it. Consider walking or shuffling the downhills to be gentler on your joints.

STAIRCLIMBING. No matter where in the world you are, you'll very likely have a flight of stairs—and an instant workout—at your disposal. Like hill running, it simulates the muscle action and power you need for climbing hills on a bike. Keep your steps quick, agile, and light, landing on and springing off the balls of your feet. Resist the urge to grab the railing and pull yourself along. Turn up the challenge by taking two steps at a time. Take it nice and easy coming back down. You can even take the elevator.

CIRCUIT TRAINING. Circuit training—strength training in a brisk fashion where you move from one exercise to the next with no rest—challenges muscles in a way they are not challenged during cycling. It strengthens the muscles you use to ride as well as the ones that support you on your bike. It also builds strength quickly while providing a cardio workout to boot. A simple circuit can be jumping jacks, squats, stepups, pushups, dips, and back extensions. Do 30 to 60 seconds of each move, repeating the entire circuit 3 times.

PUTTING IT ALL TOGETHER!

As a cyclist, you'll do all kinds of riding in your cycling life—hilly rides, flat and fast rides, slow and pleasant meanders, heck, maybe even a race (never say never). This 12-week plan was structured to help you become fit and skilled enough to handle all those types of riding. However, unlike in this program, you probably won't be doing three tempo rides one week, three hill rides the next week, and so forth. You'll be mixing them up—which is exactly what you'll be doing this week!

// **SKILL DRILL:** Rider's Choice!

Same as last week. Work on your weakness and the skills that continue to be a little shaky.

THE BYBO RIDE

TERRAIN: Mixed terrain, including flats, undulations, and inclines

Four rides this week, including the following:

* Workout from Week 6
* Workout from Week 7

* Workout from Week 8
* Rider's choice (or one long ride)

TAKE HOME: As you plan your riding weeks, use this as your model to keep your training well rounded and moving forward.

THE INSIDE RIDE

Like the outside riders, you'll be doing a large variety of workouts over your exercising life. Now, as we move into the final (!) week, we'll take a page from the outside rider's playbook and mix things up a little. So for this week we'd like you to do the following (for more Inside Ride ideas, see "Build Your Own Spin Class" on page 253):

* Workout from Week 6
* Workout from Week 7

* Workout from Week 8
* Rider's choice (or one Spin session)

TAKE HOME: As you plan your workout weeks, use this as your model to keep your training well rounded and moving forward.

BYBO CORE WORKOUT
(SEE PAGE 24 FOR EXERCISE DIRECTIONS)

Do the moves one after another like a circuit. Then repeat.

* Forearm Plank with Arm Raise
* Side Bridge Abduction

* Mountain Climbers
* Scorpion

BYBO STRETCHES
(SEE PAGE 36 FOR STRETCH DIRECTIONS)

* Figure 4
* Stork
* Windshield Wiper

* Cobra
* Prayer Pose

WORKOUT LOG

Please log your workouts for the week.

WEEK 12				
BYBO Rides (including pleasure cruise) and Core Workouts	Date: Notes:	Date: Notes:	Date: Notes:	Date: Notes:
Cross-training and/or rest	Date: Activity: Duration:	Date: Activity: Duration:	Date: Activity: Duration:	Date: Activity: Duration:

ANY OBSTACLES? _____

ACCOMPLISHMENTS? _____

OTHER NOTES: _____

BUILD YOUR OWN SPIN CLASS

The BYBO plan provided you with 12 weeks of indoor training rides. You can always go back and repeat those workouts (as you do this week). But at some point you're going to need and want new workouts to keep the gains coming and the riding feeling fresh. As an indoor cycling instructor for the past 17 years, I can tell you it's easier than you think to craft your own challenging inside ride. All you need is a playlist and a little imagination. Below you'll find samples of a couple of classic indoor cycling class structures. Add music to your liking; just try to match the tempo to the prescribed effort. It makes it easier to maintain the right exertion level.

MUSIC KEY

WARMUPS. This should be a generally up-tempo song or two that put you in the mood for exercise. Most pop or alternative rock works well here.

HILLS. Strong, steady driving beats work here. I like rap, grunge, or industrial rock.

JUMPS. A good choice is any upbeat music with a slight undulation of rhythm that feels natural to get up and down to. Swing works very well.

SPRINTS. Fast, hard-driving music of any type from metal to electronica.

COOLDOWNS. Similar to warmup music, but should bring your energy back down to chill. Electronica works well here.

BIG HILL: ABOUT 50 MINUTES

First one or two songs (5 to 10 minutes): Warm up at about 60 percent of your maximum heart rate, or MHR (exertion level 4 on a scale of 1 to 10), gradually increase the tempo so you're spinning at a high cadence with low resistance by the end of the warmup.

Next three songs (~15 minutes): Gradually increase the tension with every song to simulate a long, gradual climb. Every 2 minutes, increase the tension to very hard, get out of the saddle, and climb for 20 to 30 seconds to simulate a switchback or brief increase in incline. Exertion will be 80 to 95 percent of MHR (exertion level 7 to 9) throughout.

Next two songs (5 to 10 minutes): Gradually cool down (about 65 percent of MHR) for a few minutes. Then add a few "jumps," increasing the resistance slightly and standing to pedal for a count of 6, sitting to a count of 6, and so on, about 4 or 5 times.

Next song (~5 minutes): Sprint intervals (resistance should be like you're on a flat road). Pick up the pace for 30 seconds so you're at 90 percent of MHR (exertion level 8 or 9), then rest for 90 seconds. Repeat 3 times, taking your rest into the next song.

Final one or two songs (5 to 10 minutes): Gradually cool down, slowly decreasing your cadence. When your heart rate returns to normal, stop, dismount, and stretch.

ROLLING TERRAIN: ABOUT 50 MINUTES

First one or two songs (5 to 10 minutes): Warm up at about 60 percent of MHR (exertion level 4 on a scale of 1 to 10), gradually increase the tempo so you're spinning at a high cadence with low resistance by the end of the warmup.

Next song (~5 minutes): Increase the tension to put yourself on a big hill. Stay in the saddle for 45 seconds, get out and push hard for 15 seconds, and repeat throughout the climb.

Next song (~5 minutes): Flat-road resistance. Ride at a high cadence for 1 minute, bring it down for 1 minute, repeat.

* Next song (~5 minutes): Hill number 2. Increase the tension to put yourself on a big hill. Stay in the saddle for 45 seconds, get out and push hard for 15 seconds, and repeat throughout the climb.

* Next song (~5 minutes): Recover with an easy spin for a few minutes. Then add a few "jumps," increasing the resistance slightly and standing to pedal for a count of 6, sitting to a count of 6, and so on, about 4 or 5 times.

* Next song (~5 minutes): Sprint intervals (resistance should be like you're on a flat road). Pick up the pace for 30 seconds so you're at 90 percent of MHR (exertion level 8 or 9), rest for 90 seconds. Repeat 3 times, taking your rest into the next song.

* Next song (~5 minutes): Rolling terrain. Ride at a moderate-high cadence. Every 15 to 20 seconds, make it a click harder while maintaining your cadence (you can get out of the saddle when it gets very hard), then every 15 seconds ease the tension, still holding your pace. Repeat.

* Next song (~5 minutes): Flat-road resistance. Ride at a high cadence for 1 minute, bring it down for 1 minute, repeat.

* Last song(s): Recover and cool down, then stretch.

HIGH-INTENSITY INTERVAL MANIA

Eventually you're going to outgrow the intervals in this book and will need to go even harder if you want to keep your fitness gains and cycling speed going along an upward trajectory. That means more high-intensity interval training. When you push yourself to your absolute upper limits, everything—endurance, power, lactate threshold, efficiency, and speed—rises up and comes along for the ride, even in well-trained riders. In a study of 38 conditioned cyclists, Australian researchers found that those doing high-intensity interval training twice a week slashed their 40-K time-trial time by nearly 3 minutes (about 5 percent) and improved their average speed by nearly 1 mile per hour.

"We know even highly trained riders can increase their stroke volume [how much blood the heart pumps per beat], increase the delivery of oxygen and nutrients to muscles, and improve the muscles' ability to extract oxygen," the study author and exercise physiologist Paul Laursen, PhD, told me during an interview for *Bicycling* magazine. Intervals also seem to make your powerful sprint-centric fast-twitch fibers become more fatigue resistant, so they behave more like slow-twitch fibers, allowing you to go really fast longer.

The beauty of this kind of training is that although it's kind of painful, you don't need to do much to reap great gains. Even the shortest bouts—just 20- to 30-second micro-intervals—have been shown to increase max VO_2 (the maximum amount of oxygen your body can use during all-out exertion), improve fat burning, and boost endurance performance. And they work fast. "Just 2 weeks of training can enhance performance," says Laursen. Here are the best short workouts for all your riding needs. For each interval session, warm up for at least 5 minutes. Cool down as needed when you're done. Do these no more than twice a week, preferably midweek if you're riding long and/or hard on the weekends. "Intervals are a potent stimulus for rapid improvements. But too many per week can rapidly lead to signs of overtraining," says Laursen.

TO HANG WITH THE FAST PACK: ATTACK INTERVALS

Three to 5 minutes is the optimum interval time for raising your threshold pace. Ride as hard as you can (95 to 100 percent of MHR) for 3 minutes. Recover at an easy pace for 2 minutes. Repeat 2 or 3 times to start. Work up to 8 (very tough). Then increase the interval time.

BUILD POWER FAST: TABATA INTERVALS

Named after exercise scientist Izumi Tabata, these eye-popping efforts train your body to recruit maximum muscle fibers and fire them faster, as well as raise your lactate threshold. They take only 10 to 12 minutes. After a warmup, sprint as hard as possible (you're going for maximum wattage) for 20 seconds. Stop and coast for 10 seconds only. Repeat 6 to 8 times.

PACK A PUNCH: FLYING 40S

These slightly longer micro-intervals build power and train your body to recover quickly between hard pushes. They are helpful if you ride with a group that likes to push the pace on climbs and sprint for signs. In a medium to large gear, push as hard as you can for 40 seconds. Recover for 20 seconds. Repeat 10 times. Rest 5 minutes. Do 2 or 3 more sets.

FOR MONSTER CLIMBING: HILL CHARGES

Climbing hills builds strength. To get speed, you need to turn that strength to power (i.e., push that same gear faster). These charges do the trick. On a moderate incline that takes about 30 seconds to climb, stand out of the saddle and charge up the hill as fast as possible. Coast back down. Repeat, this time staying seated. Alternate between standing and seated for six climbs. Recover for 10 minutes. Do another set.

QUICKEN YOUR CADENCE: "10 SPEEDS"

These lightning-fast efforts demand fluid, fast feet. Over time, that silky, high-speed cadence will become second nature. Using a gear you can push at 90 to 110 rpm with effort, pedal as hard as you can for 10 seconds. Spin easy for 20 seconds. Repeat for 10 to 15 minutes. Rest 5 minutes. Do another set.

THE RIDE YOU WANT
(IN THE TIME YOU HAVE)

In an ideal world, we'd all be able to find time to do the ride we want. However, most of us live in the real world, where we need to fit our rides into designated slots of free time. Well, with careful planning you can have the best of both worlds simply by making the most of the time you have. Here's a look at how you can accomplish any number of riding goals when you have an hour—give or take—to ride.

IF YOU HAVE 30 TO 45 MINUTES

// WORKOUT 1: 30-SECOND BLASTS

Warm up for 10 minutes. Then sprint all-out for 30 seconds. Recover by spinning easy for $2^{1}/_{2}$ minutes. Repeat for as many times as you can in the time you have (12 is ideal). Cool down with a couple of minutes of easy spinning and you're done. This workout may not seem like much, but it's strong medicine, so don't do it on back-to-back days or more than twice a week.

THE BENEFIT. Research shows that even seasoned cyclists can improve their max VO_2 by 3 percent and 40-K time-trial speed by more than 4 percent in just 4 weeks by doing sets of 30-second all-out intervals.

// WORKOUT 2: SPIN-UPS

Ride at your normal cadence for 5 minutes. Then shift into a smaller gear and spin up to as fast a cadence as possible while keeping your upper body still and your pedal stroke smooth. The moment you start bouncing on the saddle, dial it back to stay controlled. Maintain that cadence for 1 minute. Recover for 3 minutes. Repeat for a total of 6 to 8 intervals and then cool down. As the effort feels easier, increase the duration of the fast spins and decrease the recovery.

THE BENEFIT. Increasing your natural cadence can improve your efficiency by shifting some of your effort from your easily fatigued leg muscles to your more resilient cardiovascular system. If you're typically a big-gear jammer, it will take some time before a higher cadence feels right. Short rides are the perfect time to practice.

// WORKOUT 3: NEIGHBORHOOD RAMBLE

When's the last time you totally unplugged, tossed a leg over your bike, and rode like a kid? Yeah, we thought so. Leave the bike computers, agendas, and padded shorts behind, jump on a bike—any bike—and ride to the post office, the park, wherever you want or need to go. Enjoy the feeling of the air on your skin, the lawn ornaments in your neighborhood, and the sights and sounds of your local rec path.

THE BENEFIT. Easy movement without effort will loosen your legs, help your body recover from previous hard efforts, and make you feel happy and recharged.

IF YOU HAVE 45 TO 60 MINUTES

// WORKOUT 1: THE TRIPLE THREAT

Warm up for 15 minutes. Crank up your intensity until you're working very hard (a 9 on a scale of 1 to 10). Hold that intensity for 3 minutes. Recover for 3 minutes. Repeat 2 more times. Finish your ride at a moderate pace, including a cooldown.

THE BENEFIT. Your max VO$_2$ is your fitness ceiling. To raise that roof, you need to do lung-searing efforts like these that force your body to find ways to increase oxygen capacity.

// WORKOUT 2: HILL ATTACKS

There are two ways to do this workout. The first way is standard hill repeats. Warm up for 10 to 15 minutes. Find a hill that takes about 5 minutes to climb and ascend it hard, staying at your maximum sustainable pace, or threshold (about a 7 effort on a scale of 1 to 10). Descend as you recover for 3 minutes. Repeat for a total of 3 to 5 times. Cool down. Or, take a more organic approach and map a 10- to 15-mile route that includes four to six good climbs. Hit the hills hard and ride moderately between efforts.

THE BENEFIT. You know the mantra: Hills make you stronger. It's true.

// WORKOUT 3: CROSS THE THRESHOLD

Warm up for 10 to 15 minutes. Increase your effort until you hit the point where you're above your comfort zone (about an 8 on your rate of perceived exertion, or RPE), and hold that for 5 to 6 minutes. Then back off and ride just below your threshold point (RPE 6) for 5 minutes. Repeat for a total of 3 or 4 times. You should be starting the next above-threshold interval before feeling fully recovered. Then cool down.

THE BENEFIT. Your threshold, the point at which your body starts producing more lactate than you can absorb, is your maximum sustainable effort. With a high threshold, you can ride really hard, really long before your legs scream at you to back off. To raise your threshold, you need to get comfortable working above that level.

IF YOU HAVE 60 TO 75 MINUTES

// WORKOUT 1: TEMPO TRAINING

Warm up for about 10 minutes. Increase your effort to a pace where you're working hard but could sustain it for a 40-K race (RPE of about 7 or 8). Hold on for 15 minutes without faltering. Pedal easy to recover for 3 minutes. Repeat 2 more times. Cool down. As you become more fit, you can increase the tempo time and decrease the recovery time until you are at tempo for a full hour.

THE BENEFIT. Any rider with two working crankarms can ride hard—for a while. But successful cyclists not only have the necessary power to climb a hill or bridge a gap, but also can sustain that kind of high-level effort.

Tempo intervals train your body to clear lactate at higher intensities so they increase your threshold and boost your sustainable "race pace." An hour or so is all you need.

// WORKOUT 2: ADULT RECESS

Find a few friends who can sneak away (your lunch hour at work is of ideal duration) and practice your pack riding skills, pacelines, and town-sign sprints.

THE BENEFIT. Time spent riding with a small group will hone your balance and riding skills, your drafting ability, and your group race tactics. Plus, it's darn fun.

// WORKOUT 3: STEADY STATE

Just as the name implies, steady-state rides maintain a consistent, unwavering effort. Though the overall intensity is only moderately hard (RPE 6), it is surprisingly difficult for many riders to sustain. Your pace should be such that you're breathing moderately and breaking a sweat, but your legs shouldn't burn. Hold it for the duration of the ride.

THE BENEFIT. Doing steady-state efforts for an hour or more improves your body's ability to tap into stored body fat as a fuel source, which improves endurance by reducing your reliance on stored carbs or glycogen stores, a limited resource. As you get fitter, you'll ride longer and more comfortably without fading or bonking, and your steady-state pace will get faster.

ROLL ON WITH THE SOCIAL MEDIA REVOLUTION

Social media can be a highly motivating force. Simply posting your daily ride goals on Facebook or tweeting them on Twitter can be enough to get you out the door. You also get the benefit of having your friends "like" what you're up to and offering words of encouragement.

You also can join or start a ride group of your own. When I came out with the book *Ride Your Way Lean*, a few readers got the notion to start a Facebook support group where they could ask each other questions, post their results, and generally seek advice and motivation. I can't wait to see similar groups using *Bike Your Butt Off!*, and I am excited about chiming in and offering support along the way.

For those who love tracking their progress and seeing how it stacks up against their past performance, as well as the performance of others, there's Strava. Strava is a bit like Facebook for cyclists and runners. You just need a GPS-enabled device to play along. Simply record your ride and plug the device into your computer when you're done to upload it to Strava's Web site. The site will provide you with a wealth of information, including distance, ride time, average speed, and maximum speed. What's more, Strava users can create special segments on any given road—usually they're climbs, but they can also be fast straightaways or descents—that Strava will automatically rank you on. So if you're the fastest local cyclist going up a particular climb, you get a little crown that stands for KOM (king of the mountain) or QOM (queen of the mountain). As with Twitter, you can follow other Strava users, and they can follow you. Like-minded riders can create private Strava groups (there's a *Ride Your Way Lean* one on there, too).

Finally, there's no lack of training and coaching apps and Web sites that provide basic workout logging and coaching tips for free or more advanced ones for a fee. Try Bicycling.com, Active.com, and TrainingPeaks.com to get started.

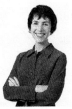

BIKE YOUR BUTT OFF! EATING PLAN: KEEP THE WEIGHT LOSS COMING

Wow, here you are. You've done it—you rode, you learned, and you've improved. Whether you are riding faster, longer, and stronger, or eating less, better, and slower (hopefully all of the above!), you have made some changes over these past 12 weeks. Even though this is the last chapter, it is only the introduction to a healthier you.

During the past 12 weeks I've discussed food choices and eating habits. Anyone can change what is on their plate or in their bowl, glass, or water bottle, but habits take longer to change, and I would expect that you have found that to be the case.

So let's do a week-by-week recap of eating goals, noting the changes you've made. What stuck? What didn't? What do you want to work harder on to turn it into a habit?

WEEK 1: We talked about food logging and creating awareness.

- How have you done with that?
- What have you learned from logging?

WEEK 2: We set your calorie goal and addressed changing your eating environment and what to buy.

- How has the calorie goal worked for you?
- What have you changed about your eating environment?
- What have you added to (or removed from) your shopping list?

WEEK 3: You ranked your hunger and learned to listen to cues and set a number of meals.

- Are you still eating according to hunger?

- How do you tune in to your internal eating cues?

- What works in terms of number of meals per day?

WEEK 4: The focus was accountability, portions at home, and eating out.

- How were you able to change your portions?

- What has changed when you eat out?

- How will you keep yourself accountable now that the program is finished?

WEEK 5: We identified and dealt with hidden saboteurs, as well as addressing fueling and hydration on the bike, caffeine, and sodium.

- What were your "aha moments"?

- What foods have you found work best when you ride?

- How have you gotten more sodium smart?

WEEK 6: We talked about the importance of protein—types, timing, and amounts—as well as recovery eating and anti-inflammatory foods.

- How have you been able to add more protein to your meals and snacks?

- What foods are you choosing to help with inflammation?

- Do you feel recovered after your hard rides? If not, why not?

WEEK 7: The goal was broadening food choices through trying new tastes and food preparation methods.

- Any new meal preparation and/or food choice ideas that you've made routine?
- Have you added any new seasonings?
- Have you discovered new kitchen gadgets?

WEEK 8: We addressed hydration and eating for bone and joint health.

- What have you done to optimize hydration?
- How do you stay hydrated on rides?
- What foods have you added for your bones and joints?

WEEK 9: We looked at rate of eating, preparing for your rides, and eating for endurance.

- Have you put the brakes on your eating speed?
- What are you eating before rides?
- What are you carrying with you so you don't bonk? (Or have you bonked? Why?)

WEEK 10: The focus was dietary fiber, adding color, eating real food, and handling special occasions.

- How have you added more fiber to your day?
- What has worked to color up the plate?
- Are you choosing items
- from the fridge more than relying on prepackaged bars?
- What are your strategies for dealing with the holidays?

WEEK 11: We took on cravings, snacks, correct portions, postride eating, and carb choices.

- What strategies have worked for dealing with cravings?

- What snack-choice changes have you made?

- What types of foods are your go-to choices after a ride?

- How have your carb choices changed in their type, amount, and/or timing?

Okay, that was an interrogation. It wasn't meant to be, but I want you to reflect on the past 3 months and ask yourself the following questions:

- What eating habits and food choices was I able to change?

- What didn't work so well?

- What do I want to focus on now to continue to reach my health and performance goals?

You don't have to change everything, and at this point, you should focus on the areas that need tweaking. Overhauling is never effective. Rather, making one small change at a time as you move forward will keep the momentum going.

I am a big fan of periodic monitoring. We all get a little cocky or complacent. Writing things down occasionally is the reality check you need to affirm you are really doing what you need to be doing or confirm that you could be doing better.

Also share your journey with others! As Selene mentioned earlier when discussing Strava and such, social media can be a powerful motivational tool. Blog, tweet, post on Facebook—let others know what you have done. You can be an inspiration. Plus, when you put yourself in the spotlight, you feel more obligated to carry through. Take pictures of your food; use Pinterest to post a great recipe; if you see a new product in the grocery store, snap it, buy it, and share. What a great way to reinforce the positive and motivate others!

FINAL WORDS
GOING INTO THE LAST MILE

You have asked your body and brain to do a lot these past 12 weeks. What has changed about your body? Are you fitter, leaner, lighter? If so, remember that if you now weigh less than you did when you started, your body actually needs fewer calories at this lighter weight. If you want to keep the weight loss coming, you may want to recalculate your calorie needs based on your current weight.

If you did not change much during the past 3 months, view yourself as a work in progress. Try to identify a few strategies you may have skipped or skimmed over the first time around that may help you achieve your goals.

Above all, continue to seek support, take care of your body, and congratulate yourself for becoming a healthier you.

Secrets of Their Success

SHERRIE ZACKER, 45

WEIGHT LOST:
1 pound, plus ½ inch off her waist

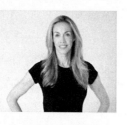

Sherrie had one goal when she came to us about joining the BYBO plan. She wanted to be able to ride her bike. You can find details of her tales of newbie cycling woes on page 220, but in a nutshell, she was a self-described disaster on wheels, nearly swerving into other riders, pedaling like mad, unable to shift, toppling over at stop signs, you name it. Unfortunately, like so many riders who are new to the sport, she blamed herself for her inability to ride competently and confidently and racked her bike for what she thought was for good in her garage.

Then she heard about the BYBO plan. "I would love to be a part of it," she said. I agreed and met her to give her the plan and the details. Before I could leave, she cornered me. "Okay, I'm sure you'll cover this, but how do you shift?" I gave her the basics and assured her she would get everything she needed in a step-by-step fashion. Over the course of the plan, Sherrie simply soared.

"I have been riding and absolutely loving it. I'm out there at least three times a week and learning so much from the drills, lessons, and interval training. I feel the training in places in my body where I don't normally feel it when I do indoor cycling, and I love that. I am getting much more confident on the bike outdoors and many of my fears (i.e., navigating an intersection with traffic lights and traffic, falling over because I'm clipped in, riding in the rain, etc.) are going away and not holding me back. As I've mentioned, all the BYBO workouts and practice have really helped me master what I thought I'd never get right. Starting, stopping, scanning for traffic seems so basic, but it was a great way to start. I finally understand how to shift gears. THANK YOU! Shifting before getting to the point where I needed to was also very helpful."

There are still some sticky spots for Sherrie, but she's happy to be conquering them one by one. "I need more practice steering the bike with my body—I can't help but feel like I'm going to fall over—but I'll get there. I'm glad you encouraged me to take on the hills. I was avoiding them. I did have to get off and walk once or twice, but I got farther every time. Pushing the bike forward before returning to the seat was brilliant for me. Pushing down and pulling up while I pedaled was a much-needed reminder. I still need to work on my speed. But it's all coming along!"

On the eating front, Sherrie chose her foods wisely. She just was not as wise in choosing when to eat. Though Sherrie was already at a healthy, fit weight, she did want to get control of her eating habits to prevent the small swings on the scale that had become the norm. "I thought I had a pretty good diet going, but I learned so much. I learned to eat slower, incorporate 'no-eating zones' like at work and in front of the computer. Now I sit and enjoy my food in a relaxing way. I learned to eat full meals so I don't get hungry and snack or graze. No wonder I had such a hard time with my food diaries, I was eating constantly and mindlessly. For anyone who has trouble with their weight or eating, I recommend trying to record your diet as recommended in this plan. It helped me stop eating everywhere all the time!

"Thank you for being the inspiration I needed to get on the road with my bike. I now have confidence on my bike because I've learned the fundamentals. In fact, I've even taught my cycling friends a thing or two."

INDEX

Underscored page references indicate sidebars and tables.
Boldface references indicate photographs and illustrations.

C

Cadence
  brisk, 43, 91–92
  decreasing, for power transfer, 193
  for hip pain relief, 177
  improving, 92–94
    workouts for, 94–96
  on mountain bike trails, 125–26
  in spin-up workout, 258–59
Caffeine, 118–19, 179
Calorie burning, factors increasing
  basal metabolic rate, 57, 57
  cycling, ix, xvii, 51
  fiber, 211
  intervals, xiv
  non-exercise activity thermogenesis, 58
  riding off road, 126
  standing, 203
Calorie deficit, for weight loss, 52, 58, 267
Calorie intake, tracking, 59, 62
Calories, in beverages, 115
Calves, foam rolling, 169, **169**
Cancer
  preventing, ix, 137
  sitting increasing risk of, 202
Capillaries, leg, cycling increasing, xiii
Carbloading, 198
Carbohydrates
  choices of, 85, 236–37
  for endurance rides, 198–99
  protein and, 121, 134–35, 141
  during rides, 116–17, 234–35
Cardioresistance training, in Inside
      Rides, 19, 56, 78, 96, 112, 131, 152, 209
Cassette, 10, **11**, 43
Century ride, readiness for, 146
Chafing, 44, 247
Chain, after-rain care of, 128
Chain lube, 45, 50, 128
Chainrings, 10, **11**, 43, 44
Chamois Butt'r, 44, 247

Charity rides, 144, 146, 147, 244
Cholesterol, fiber lowering, 211, 212
Circles, in turning skill drill, 76
Circuit training, 249
Climbing hills. *See* Hill climbing
Clipless pedals, 11, 72–73, 93, 110, 190, 221, 222
Clothing, cycling, 104
  compression wear, 167
  layering, 64, 188–90
  location for storing, 12, 206
  for longer rides, 72–74
  recommended, 8–9, 108–9
  for riding in rain, 127
  for visibility, 90
Cobra stretch, 39, **39**
Coffee, 119
Cold treatments, for recovery, 167
Colorful foods, 213
Commuting by bike, 12, 146, 244–47
Compression wear, 167
Computer, cycling, 74
Core
  bracing, during hill climbing, 148–49
  protecting, in rain, 127
  strengthening, 241 (*see also* BYBO Core Workout)
Cornering, 68, 69–70, 128, 150
Coronary heart disease, cycling preventing, xiv
Cortisol, cycling reducing, xvi
Countersteering, 69
Countertop grill, 13
Courtesy, 90
Crank plank (Core Move), 28, **28**
Cranks, 11, **11**
Crashes. *See* Accidents
Cravings, 231–32
Cross the threshold workout, 260
Cross-training activities, 248–49
Cruisers, 6, **6**
Cycling
  calorie burning from, ix, xvii, 51
  current popularity of, xii
  enjoyment from, 68

S